KETO DIET AND INTERMITTENT FASTING FOR BEGINNERS

Your NEW 21-Day Meal Plan to Lose Weight, Heal Your Body, and Nourish Your Mind. Be MORE CONFIDENT AND STRONGER by Living a Ketogenic Lifestyle NOW!

By reading this document, the reader agrees that under no circumstances is the author responsible for any losses, direct or indirect, which are incurred as a result of the use of the information contained within this document, including, but not limited to, — errors, omissions, or inaccuracies.

Table of Contents

Introduction

Considering you are reading this book, it is safe to say that you want to shed off some extra pounds that you may have. You may not like your current appearance, want to fit in some clothes for a special occasion, or you just want to get healthy, whatever the case, this is the right book for you. As weight loss is not a new issue, there have been various approaches to it. If you have been looking around for fast weight loss regimens, then there is a high chance that you have come across the words 'intermittent fasting' and 'ketogenic diet.'

The most generic advice that people give for weight loss is to eat a lot of whole-grain carbohydrates and keep away from saturated fat as if it is taboo. Do you know that it is all a lie? Your body needs fat, and it is actually the main component of the ketogenic diet, and it contributes to most of the calories in the diet.

Intermittent fasting is another weapon you should have in your arsenal that can make you get a fair chance to fight against excess fat. It has been used across the ages in different societies all around the world. It is even an integral part of many religions and cultures as it helps clear your mind and clear toxins that have accumulated in your body.

These approaches to burn fat have gained a lot of popularity due to the ease of doing them and their effectiveness in burning fat. Movie stars, athletes, and even regular people use them as ways to keep their weight in check. However, people do not have a lot of information on them; they have vague ideas, which makes them derive false conclusions that are not backed up by facts.

To clarify things, even before diving right into the information in this book, it is best to understand the difference between IF and the keto diet. Suppose it is not a diet but a meal planner that is designed to enhance weight loss, among other health advantages. In that case, the keto diet is a diet that highly restricts carbohydrates and increases the amount of fat that you take to be fuller for longer and be able to make fat your main energy source amid other advantages that will be discussed later on.

Inside this book, you will find a vast amount of information about IF and the ketogenic diet. You will know why and how they work so well and how they can work together to enhance your weight loss experience. You will also know about their benefits and downsides, and directions are as safe as you practice them.

Everyone wants to lose weight, but not everyone wants to go through the challenges that the process of weight loss entails.

It's one thing to put your body through the struggles of strenuous exercise, but following a restrictive diet can be challenging for most of us.

Perhaps you've been disappointed by diet plans that have come and gone without results. Maybe you're tired of feeling unhappy about what you see in the mirror? Maybe you just want to do what's best for your body.

Whatever your reason, the ketogenic diet might be just the answer you're looking for.

If you're fed up with putting all your effort into a weight loss plan that doesn't deliver, maybe it's time to try something new.

In this comprehensive guide, you'll learn everything you need to know about the ketogenic diet. You'll discover how it started, why it works, and how you can apply it in your life to achieve the benefits that it promises.

You can overcome these severe problems just by intermittent fasting. It is not as if problems don't have their solutions. Solutions do exist. It depends if you are willing enough to convert your problem to your advantage. Intermittent fasting is not as if you fast. You only schedule your eating habits. You only eat at the right time. You do not eat 24/7; that is the root of obesity. Constant snacking slacks you from your life.

Once you achieve your goal, you will experience the benefits yourself. If you do not, you will live in a hell created by your brain forever. Individual guilt will glue to your mental stability. Hence you need to follow your dreams.

PART ONE: KETO DIET AND INTERMITTENT FASTING

Chapter 1: What is Ketogenic Diet?

Ketogenic diet is a high-fat diet that encourages the body to produce ketones.

Initially, the keto diet was developed for individuals with epilepsy and similar seizure disorders. In the 1920s and '30s, the ketogenic diet was used as one of the cornerstones of the treatment of epilepsy in children. According to research, these molecules have the potential to manage seizures with their powerful anticonvulsant effects.

Today, the ketogenic diet has made a comeback as one of the most popular diet trends of the modern age.

Since hitting the mainstream market, the keto diet has seen unprecedented popularity. It is in the front and center as one of the most effective weight loss strategies we've seen in the last 30 years.

While being an effective diet should be reason enough for its popularity, a few other things about the keto diet make it stand out in a sea of hyped-up weight loss strategies.

The fact that the keto diet doesn't tell you to eat less fat makes it controversial - a factor that has led to the development of its cult following.

We're conditioned to think that more fat in our diet should make us more fat, but something about the way the keto diet works produces the opposite results.

With such an uncommon mechanism, the diet strategy piqued the interest of hundreds of thousands of dieters, blasting it off towards worldwide popularity.

How the Ketogenic Diet Works

On the surface, there are a few things about the ketogenic diet that are generally known to most of those who've heard of it - whether or not they've tried the method themselves.

For instance, the ketogenic diet:

It doesn't focus on caloric intake or metabolism

It encourages more fat consumption

It satisfies hunger and keeps you feeling full for longer period

It works for most body types.

These snippets aren't new. In fact, most of those who try to sell the keto diet idea will weigh down on these points to get their message across.

While it's all good and well to know what the ketogenic diet does, it's equally important to understand how the keto diet does it.

Sure, not everyone can be a physiology expert, and certainly, not everyone wants to be. But, understanding how the diet works will make it easier to pattern choices throughout the process to support this weight loss strategy's unique physiological mechanism.

Ketosis

Ketosis is a metabolic state where the body's energy needs are fulfilled by ketones rather than glucose. When you are on the keto diet, the body operates as it would in a starving mode, which means that an alternate source of energy must be obtained to keep the different cell functions operational (Leonard & Daniel, 2019). Insufficient carb consumption triggers the body to start breaking down the available fats stored in the body, which is, in the real sense, a survival mode. Since the keto diet mimics fasting/starving, the body gets into a protective state where it must keep the body's functions operational by providing an alternate energy source. When the body reaches the ketosis state, the body shifts entirely from relying on glucose as the primary energy source to the absolute reliance on ketones. The body will remain in such a state until you reintroduce carbs back to your diet, in which case glycolysis will begin once again.

Signs that you are in Ketosis

As has already been stated, keto dieters must strive to achieve ketosis so that they can witness most of the benefits. Since ketosis marks a change in the normal body's metabolic function, the changed function manifests differently. Once you reach ketosis, you are bound to realize one or more of the following signs:

The Keto Flu

The keto flu resembles the regular cold flu, and it is majorly caused by the immediate electrolyte imbalance that occurs once you begin dieting. The flu presents about a week after starting the diet, and you are likely to experience mild headaches, fatigue, extreme weakness, and pain in the muscles. For some people, the signs may be too severe to the extent that they may have a hard time functioning normally. Note that some of the electrolytes that the keto diet may be unable to provide in sufficient quantities for your body's needs include sodium, calcium, and potassium (Healthline, 2019). Some people can overlook the symptoms while others get it so rough that they experience extreme symptoms such as nausea, constipation, inability to sleep, and irritability. First, if you experience the flu, it is good news since it shows that you are on the right track. However, you do not have to be miserable, and you can opt to boost the nutrients by taking supplements.

The Keto Rash

The keto rash may occur immediately when ketosis begins to take place, but it clears on its own in a few days. Note that being a beginner on the keto diet means that your body knows only one metabolism mode: glycolysis. Once ketosis begins, the ketones may be identified as foreign objects by the body, leading to inflammation of all the cells they are transported to. The skin is among those affected, resulting in a rash. Also, people who do not take supplements are bound to experience an extreme deficiency, which shows on the skin. The keto rash is very mild and should not really bother you.

Increased Thirst

The keto diet is marred by increased dehydration as a result of an electrolyte imbalance. When you suddenly begin feeling thirstier despite the amount of water you drink, it is a sign that ketosis has already started taking place in your body.

Increased Ketones in the Body

Some people are incredibly serious about the keto diet and will take tests to confirm whether ketosis has begun taking place periodically. Usually, there are two key ways by which you can test the ketone levels in the body:

• Blood Test. Taking a blood test is one of the surest and most accurate methods of finding the ketone levels in the bloodstream, although it is also more expensive than the other methods. The blood test is conducted using a ketone meter, which works just like a regular blood test. One of the significant disadvantages of this method is that it's invasive since you have to prick your finger to get drops of blood, which you then place in the measurement meter. Most of the meters are current and digitized, thus enabling the getting of results directly into the connected computers.

• Urine Test. Urine tests are just as effective as blood tests, and the major advantage is that they are the least invasive. The urine test is straightforward as all you have to do is place ketone strips in the urine stream or dip them into a cup, and depending on the color change, you will know the levels of ketones in the body.

Benefits of Ketosis

Weight Loss

When you are on the keto diet, weight loss is imminent. One of the most common reasons why most people swear by the keto diet is the assured weight loss capabilities. Unlike most fad diets that promise weight loss and fall short of people's expectations, the keto diet is backed up by scientific evidence, which means that every person who reaches ketosis will undoubtedly lose weight.

Clearing of the Skin and the Reduction of Acne

Skin problems, particularly acne, are one of the ailments that have people spending thousands of dollars every year to treat/clear. Everybody wants to look good. Whether male or female, everyone is undoubtedly working toward becoming the best versions of themselves; one of the ways is being through the quest for clearer skin. This is no vanity in any way, and I am sure that you also want to know directions to get that bright, youthful skin.

Improved Cognitive Function

When you start following the keto diet, you will realize increased cognitive function as soon as ketosis begins to take place. Several reasons contribute to the boosted cognitive function, some of which include:

• Reduced neurological inflammation. When you start the keto diet, one of the things that you will realize almost immediately is that your brain will begin feeling much sharper. As has already been stated, the keto diet helps reduce inflammation caused by free radicals.

• Mitochondrial biogenesis. The mitochondria are organelles found in body cells, which are responsible for the production of energy. The body energy is obtained when two key ingredients are combined: oxygen and nutrients derived from food consumption. Typically, the energy is created through a distinct function known as oxidative phosphorylation in the mitochondria.

Increased Energy

Have you ever tried anything when your energy levels were at your lowest? Even simple tasks such as walking to a nearby shop can feel impossible, and you are likely to end up being the least productive and proactive. You will forget this lack of energy when you start to live a keto lifestyle.

Directions to Maximize Ketosis

Now you can enter into a state of ketosis just by lowering your carb intake. However, there are always better ways of doing the same thing, right?

Following the steps below, you will prolong the period that your body stays in ketosis, thereby increasing your ketogenic diet's effectiveness.

Keep your daily carbohydrate intake below 20g.

Keep your protein levels at around 70g per day.

Don't starve! Consume adequate levels of fat. Remember that the body is going to need fat to burn.

Try to avoid snacks and stick to your breakfast, lunch, and dinner meals with nothing in between.

The Keto Flu

The first few weeks of the keto diet can be rough. There is not only a lot of change to your day-to-day lifestyle (especially if you're someone who eats a high carb diet and you're quite simply just not used to cooking for yourself), it can also feel pretty terrible thanks to the keto flu.

Like I said before, the keto flu is something you'll probably start feeling within the first few days of the diet. You may not feel it at all. Some people manage to smoothly transition from a regular diet to a low-carb diet without any problem whatsoever. You probably won't be one of them. It can feel very similar to the flu, ergo the name "keto flu."

Symptoms include vomiting, nausea, constipation, diarrhea, headaches, irritability, stomach pain, muscle soreness, muscle weakness, sleeping difficulty, sugar cravings, muscle cramps, dizziness, and poor concentration. Typically, the keto flu will last about a week, but symptoms can last up to a month. The worst will probably happen within these seven days. This can often make first-time keto dieters throw in the towel, but you need to push through—at least for the first seven days.

On the first day, you probably won't feel much. However, you will start feeling something by the end of it, probably in the middle of the night. You will probably have a hard time sleeping and have to pee a lot. The next day you might feel as if you should just stay in bed all day, and this feeling will worsen, then get better for about a week. When you've reached that final day, which is a great accomplishment, you might feel better, but because it all depends on the person, you might still be feeling the effects.

Why does this happen? Well, think of your body almost like a house. Your house needs renovation. A big one. The wiring and plumbing are bad, your walls are not insulated, the floorboards have holes, and it's just not a good house. The keto diet is now changing out all the floorboards, properly insulating the walls, and fixing the wiring and plumbing. This will take time, and for a while, you might be sleeping in your house without walls. You have to feel worse before you feel better.

You can reduce symptoms, thankfully. Some of the methods to achieve that include:

• Drink a lot of water. The keto diet will rapidly shed water stores, and replacing these fluids can help you with symptoms such as fatigue, muscle cramping, and especially digestive issues like diarrhea and constipation.

• Avoid strenuous exercise. If you are someone who works out or plans on implementing a workout routine with your new diet, hold off for the first week or two or until you feel like the worst of the symptoms have passed. All of your body's energy is going towards remodeling your body, and it must adapt first.

Consider very light exercise, like going on walks or trying out yoga.

• Replace electrolytes. As your insulin levels decrease, your kidneys reduce and shed the number of electrolytes, such as sodium. Replace them with tablets, gel, or packs to be mixed in a drink. Just check the sugar content. They can be bought at local fitness stores or ordered online.

• Get lots of sleep. Sleep is essential if you want to be successful in any part of your life. You need a good amount of sleep. If you have issues sleeping, consider drinking lavender tea, turn off electronics like cell phones and tablets about an hour before bed, or take a bath or shower. The hot water helps relax your muscles and makes you sleepy.

The keto flu can last several weeks, with the first week being the worst. In the first week, you might find yourself wanting to quit, but do your best to just push through it. You got this. You're totally up for it.

Don't forget to celebrate when you've reached that seventh day—and not with food. Consider letting yourself do something you've wanted to do for a while, like going to see a movie that you've wanted to see or splurging on concert tickets. Something that will get you up and moving and being away from food is your best bet.

Get in Your Keto Lifestyle in Five Steps

Succeeding in the Ketogenic Diet relies not only on knowing about the right information but creating an actual diet plan.

Your action plan involves knowing about the right foods to avoid and eat and many other things.

Getting Started

There are a few ways someone can prepare their body to start the keto diet so that the change will not be a shock to their system. The first way is to start minimizing carb intake before beginning the diet in earnest. That allows your body to start adjusting to using fewer carbs for energy to be prepared for it when the supply is cut off almost entirely. Another way is to start using coconut oil when cooking. This is one of the best fats a person can embrace on keto because it contains medium-chain triglycerides (MCT), which are fats that can be transported straight to the liver and turned into energy. If the body is already accustomed to working with fat as energy, it can make the switch to keto a little easier.

Doing extra exercising before starting keto can also help to deplete extra glucose stored in the muscles, so the body is not purging such large amounts at the beginning of the diet. This will help encourage the body to reach ketosis faster when a person transitions to mostly fats. It can also be beneficial to get exercise before the keto flu (which can make some people unwilling to exercise). In tandem with working out more, though, a person should replace the lost glucose stored with healthy fats. If they can gradually prepare their body for more fats before starting in earnest, it can help the transition smoother and maybe even avoid the keto flu.

The day before someone starts the diet, they should also do a short fast to purge those last stores of glucose and get the body to start drawing on fat sources. This will promote ketosis before the diet is even started, so when a person starts eating fats, their body is already in the correct state to process them.

Finally, a keto beginner should make sure they are not neglecting their protein. Keeping enough protein in the system helps keep ketones and blood sugar levels at a healthy balance. It can also keep people from feeling too hungry between meals or serve as a great snack. Also, if someone is focusing on toning muscles, protein is a great way to promote muscle mass.

The Ketogenic Diet is a very straightforward diet regimen that you can follow. While the principle behind this diet regimen involves consuming fats, it is crucial to note that not all foods are created equally. Thus, below are the foods that you are allowed to eat under the Ketogenic Diet.

Fats and oils: This diet encourages the intake of healthy fats to drive ketosis in your body. However, there are certain amounts of fats that you should consume, and these include animal fat, butter, eggs, olive oil, sunflower oil, fatty fishes, nuts, avocado, peanut butter, and seeds.

Proteins: Proteins should be consumed moderately when following this particular diet. It is crucial to choose protein sourced from free-range, organic, or grass-fed livestock. Under this diet regimen, you can consume fish, shellfish, eggs, meat, and poultry.

Vegetables: Vegetables are encouraged in the Ketogenic Diet to include dark and leafy green vegetables as they contain high amounts of minerals but minimal amounts of carbs.

Water: To avoid dehydration, you are encouraged to drink a lot of water. However, if you want to drink other beverages, you can do so as long as they are not alcoholic and unsweetened.

Sweeteners: Sweeteners can also be consumed but make sure that they are sugar-free. Go for liquid sweeteners as they do not contain any carbohydrate binders such as maltodextrin or dextrose. You can try stevia, sucralose, and erythritol.

What Food to Avoid

Like other weight-loss diets, the Ketogenic Diet is also restrictive to certain types of foods, particularly those containing high amounts of carbohydrates. But other than carb-laden foods, there are other foods that you should avoid if you are going to follow the Ketogenic Diet.

Fruits: Although fruits are healthy, the Ketogenic Diet discourages fruits' consumption as they contain high amounts of sugar – fructose.

Processed foods: Processed foods contain high amounts of sugar as well as trans-fat. Trans fat is a bad type of fat that should be avoided at all costs.

Root vegetables: Root vegetables such as potatoes, beetroot, and carrots, to name a few, contain high amounts of carbohydrates.

Keto Diet Pantry Stock and Store Cupboard

When it comes to shopping for your ingredients, you must stock up on keto-friendly ingredients. The best thing about your ketogenic pantry is that ingredients are now easily available from your local food stores. Make sure that your ingredients are fresh, and opt for those that are not processed. Below are some of the food items that you need to stock up on in your pantry.

Low-Carb Vegetables: Stock up on low-carb vegetables such as spinach, arugula, mushrooms, cauliflower, broccoli, kale, cabbages, zucchini, and bell peppers. Not only do they contain fewer carbs, but they are also high in fibers, vitamins, and minerals.

Low Sugar Fruits: You can still enjoy fruits as there are fruits that are low in carbs. These include citrus fruits, avocado, blackberries, blueberries, and strawberries. Stay away from bananas, pineapples, apples, papaya, grapes, and pears.

Seafood: Seafood is a good source of fats as well as high-quality proteins. Stock up on wild salmon, sardines, mackerel, crab, shrimps, tuna, and mussels. Avoid anything that is farmed and opt for wild-caught seafood.

Meat, Poultry, And Eggs: Stock up on fatty meats, turkey, venison, chicken, and beef as long as they are organic and grass-fed.

Nuts and Seeds: Nuts and seeds are good sources of fats. You can stock up on peanuts, walnuts, sesame seeds, Macadamia nuts, Brazil nuts, chia seeds, almonds, pumpkin seeds, and many others.

Dairy Products: Dairy products such as cottage cheese, plain Greek yogurt, butter, and cream are high in fat but make sure that they are not made with any form of sugar.

Oils: Oils from fruits and nuts are good for the body. Opt for healthy oils sourced from coconut butter, olive oil, avocado oil, nut oil, and MCT oil.

Keto Approved Condiments: Keto-approved condiments such as olive oil mayonnaise, mustard, and oil-based salad dressing that are not highly processed and do not come with added sugar.

Keto Approved Snacks: keto-approved snacks such as nut butter, sugar-free jerky, dried seaweeds, nuts, and low-carb crackers are approved for this particular diet.

Chocolate: As long as you consume dark chocolates, then this is approved for the Ketogenic Diet.

The Guide to Keto Diet Meal Plan

When it comes to starting with this particular diet, you must create a meal plan. But the Keto Diet meal plan does involve not only planning your meals way ahead of time but also other things. Below are the things that you need to do in order to be successful while following the Ketogenic Diet.

Cut The Worst Carbs Out Of Your Diet: The first thing you need to do is do an inventory of the foods you consume. Once you have already created an inventory, the next thing to do is to cut the worst carbs out of your diet completely. These include sweets, bread, pastries, snacks, and many others.

Try Some Light Exercise: Exercising is very important if you want to push your body to ketosis faster. Exercises allow the body to use up the free glucose in your bloodstream so that you can switch on ketosis.

Don't Ignore Your Macros: The dietary macronutrients for this particular diet is divided into 60% fats, 35% proteins, and 5% carbohydrates. Moreover, a dieter needs to consume no more than 2000 kcal per day, and that the carbohydrates should be kept at a minimum consumption of 20 grams per day.

Don't Skimp On Protein: Protein is important for muscle building, so don't skimp on them when following this diet. However, make sure that you choose the right protein choices. Ideally, you need to consume lean and organic meats sourced from grass-fed livestock.

Do Not Obsess Over Your Ketone Levels: When you are still starting with the Ketogenic Diet, you mustn't obsess over your ketone levels. Whether your ketone levels are high or low, what matters is that you achieve ketosis.

Your Body Reaction to The Meal Plan Along the Way
The increasing levels of ketone bodies in the body due to ketosis can affect the body. The collection of the symptoms and side effects is called the Keto Flu. Below are the things that you will expect if you follow the Ketogenic Diet.

Weight Loss: The most evident reaction to following the Ketogenic Diet is weight loss within a few days following the diet.

Thirst: Many people who follow the ketogenic diet feel thirstier than usual due to water loss. High levels of ketone bodies can lead to dehydration as well as electrolyte imbalance, so be sure that you drink a lot of water.

Muscle Cramps and Spasms: Because it is easy for people following the Ketogenic Diet to become dehydrated, muscle cramps and spasms may be common side effects due to electrolyte imbalance.

Headaches: Headaches can be common side effects once you switch to this diet regimen. It can happen due to the consumption of fewer carbs. However, the side effects usually last for only a few days after starting the diet.

Fatigue and Weakness: During the ketogenic diet's initial stages, you might feel tired and weaker than usual. This happens because the body is still adjusting after making the switch to a low carb diet.

Stomach Upset: Making any changes to your diet can increase the risk of digestive complaints. To reduce the risk, make sure that you drink plenty of liquid.

Disrupted Sleep: Disrupted sleep is a common side effect among people who switch to the ketogenic diet. However, this side effect usually goes away after a few weeks.

Bad Breath: Bad breath is a common side effect due to ketosis. As the ketone bodies leave the body, it produces a certain type of smell. If the body's ketone body is acetone, then the breath can smell fruity or sweet. However, acetophenone and BHB can contribute to bad breath.

Better Concentration: As the symptoms fade over time, most people notice that they have better concentration following the ketogenic diet.

Pushing Forward

Eliminating an entire food group from a person's diet is a big change and can take some time to get used to. The key to making it through this major adjustment is to plan accordingly and be familiar with what the process will look and feel like.

Someone looking to start keto and quit grains should first pick a time when no other stressful things are happening in their life. This can help them weather keto's side effects and lose a fuel source without added pressures that might convince them to cheat on the diet before they get started. Additionally, a person typically feels fatigued and rundown during the adjustment period. During this time, it can be beneficial not to push the body by doing any high-intensity exercise instead of focusing on low-impact activities that don't stress the body.

Keeping hydrated can also help replenish the nutrients that muscles and organs are losing during the detox period. Insulin levels usually drop when a person cuts out grains because the body has fewer sugars to process. By increasing salt intake and drinking water, a person can keep insulin levels closer to their normal range and feel less of the drop's effects.

A person should also be prepared for cravings because they will come, and they will likely be intense. They can take precautions beforehand by cleaning out their pantry and stocking it with treats that do not contain grains, such as dried fruit or healthy fats. Having things to curb hunger can help curb the cravings as well. This is also a time when a person can embrace substitutes. At first, many substitutes can seem strange and unsatisfying because they have a different structure or texture than the original. If a person can accept this as what is approved, though, then over time, their palate will adjust, and they might even come to love their grain substitutes.

With the wide variety of foods and food substitutes available today, plenty of dairy and grain substitutes are keto-approved or designed specifically for people on keto. This can help make the transition a little easier for people who might be nervous about giving up their daily sandwich.

The first simple step is to trade in the bleached flour for nut flours such as almond or coconut flour. However, it is important to keep in mind that these flours will not act the same way as regular flour when a person is cooking with them. They do not rise or moisten the same as traditional flour, so some adjustments are usually needed in recipes. Another easy fix is to substitute keto-approved natural sweeteners if a person is having trouble staying away from sweets. People can reach for natural options such as stevia or monk fruit sweetener to satisfy their sweet tooth and stay in ketosis.

Some people find it difficult to leave starches behind, such as the various forms of cooked potatoes. There are a wide variety of low-carb veggies that can take a potato's place. Think radishes for a potato-like consistency, or switch it up with tomatoes, eggplant, artichoke, or onions. If rice is proving to be problematic, someone can take a cauliflower's head and make a great substitute. Simply placing cauliflower florets in a food processor can make cauliflower rice, which can be used just like regular rice but packs twice the benefits.

Pasta can be replaced with spiralized veggies, which are growing in fame. Zucchini, squash, and even carrot noodles are growing more and more popular in grocery stores and can be surprisingly easy to find. A person can also invest in a spiralizer to make their noodles at home or focus on spaghetti squash, which only needs to be scraped out after roasting to obtain a large portion of veggie noodles.

Chapter 2: What is Intermittent Fasting

Intermittent Fasting is essentially the practice of restricting mealtimes, reducing snacking, or cutting out days of eating, based on the method one chooses. One of the most popular IF methods is 5:2, which is to eat five days a week and fast the other two. Others focus on eating windows and fasting periods within each day. The easiest method to start with for IF, however, is just to stop eating snacks.

So many of us snack unconsciously or when we're getting moody without any real hunger. Many of us eat unconsciously in general, and then we're confused about why our bodies hold onto the weight. Intermittent Fasting reminds the body what food is for, and it restarts that nutritional absorption potential. All you have to do is cut out the snacks, fast a few hours a day, or just drink water a few days a week.

IF is both a dietary choice and a lifestyle, but those who have the most success with IF will tell you that it instantly became a lifestyle for them. Sure, dieting plans and IF can match up nicely, but for some, IF requires no dietary change whatsoever. The point is to eat less and to eat less often. The brain and the body will respond in no time.

How it Works

It gives the body a break and provides a moment to recalibrate. And with this recalibration, neurotransmitters are released easier in the brain, and one's senses of hungry and full are adjusted back to how they should be. Once the food is eaten after the fast, too, nutritional absorption is boosted throughout the entire body to benefit one's organs.

Additionally, Intermittent Fasting recalibrates one's hormones in relation to stress and hunger so that balanced mood, patience, and intellect can be increased despite the seeming lack of food. IF tells the brain and body to restart. It makes your system go back to basics and clean out any gunk, and a lot of that gunk tends to be stored fat or water weight. It sees the toxins in your body and refuses to let you hold onto them. Overall, IF proves that a change in routine can have great and lasting effects on one's health.

Intermittent Fasting takes off the unwanted load from your internal system. It helps your body in regrouping its strength. Your vital organs get a chance to become more sensitive to responses. All this can happen by simply practicing extended fasting periods in your daily routine.

Excess of things to eat is a major cause of problems in the body. We are keeping our bodies under the constant pressure of work. Eating and drinking may look like a fulfilling exercise, but it is a task for the body to process. This task keeps the body engaged and doesn't give it the time to relax. This leads to fatigue, and various body functions will start developing a kind of resistance.

To understand it in simple words, you can take the analogy of cooking something in your kitchen. Let us suppose you have started boiling pasta. Pasta boils in a definite period. Neither overcooked pasta is good for eating nor the uncooked one. Now suppose you start cooking pasta and add some more to the same water after 2 minutes. You wait for 2 minutes and add some more. You keep adding more and more pasta after 2 minutes. In the end, you would have a mess at your hand. Some of the pasta that was added in the beginning would get overcooked. Some of it would get cooked fairly, while most of it would remain undercooked. You would have an unedible pasta on your plate, although you boiled it for the desired period and followed the process thoroughly.

We are doing exactly the same with our bodies. Any specific meal, howsoever insignificant in quantity and light in nature, takes a few hours to get digested properly. Experts believe that food takes at least 6-8 hours to pass through our stomach and the small intestine. From here, the process gets very slow, and the food gets absorbed very slowly. So our body needs longer gaps between meals to process the food properly and absorb all the nutrients. However, we are not giving this time to our body, and this is the cause of most problems.

When we start our day, we start by breakfast or an early morning snack, which happens between 7 and 9 am. Between 11-12, people will take snacks and tea again. This is a meal right before lunch, which takes place between 1–3 pm. The lunch causes lethargy in most people, and hence tea and beverages come to the rescue. Many people also prefer the evening snacks between 5–6 pm as this allows them to have late dinner and helps eliminate hunger. The last meal of the day takes place ideally between 9–11 pm, right before bedtime.

This whole routine doesn't give your body any time to relax. Your digestive system is always at work. It never gets those 6-8 hours to process a meal before the next one comes completely. You are simply adding more and more pasta to the same pot and spoiling the whole meal.

The food in our gut is not getting processed properly as our gut holds food items at various stages of processing that get the same treatment. This causes most of the digestive issues. Your body fails to absorb the required nutrients, and you have no other options than to take nutrient supplements.

Your insulin levels always remain very high as frequent meals keep spiking blood glucose levels.

Your hunger and satiety hormones start responding in a wacky manner as the differentiation gets difficult.

You get prone to diabetes, and insulin resistance in your body increases with time.

It also leads to an increase in your blood pressure and insulin resistance trips other vital parameters.

From chronic inflammation to the overactive release of stress hormones, the body is in a continuous struggle.

All this can happen simply because you choose to eat whenever you liked.

Now, imagine that you have been doing that for your whole life. Until the body is in a teenage stage, it has a very powerful digestive mechanism, and there is a constant release of growth hormones. There is a high energy need, and hence this doesn't affect us much, and there is no significant weight gain. But, once you cross teenage stage and start leading a bit sedentary life, obesity starts kicking in. The digestive process starts getting weak, and all the metabolic functions come under great strain.

The first thing intermittent fasting does is that it strengthens your digestive process by reducing the pressure from it. It gives your crucial insulin formation functions, the desired break, and your system can relax. It is also the system that affects your fat storage, and hence your fat-burning begins.

Getting Started

So, we've made it. We stand now with enough valuable information and proper preparation for setting a date to start including Intermittent Fasting in our daily lives. This does not mean that we have to fast every day, but fasting is on our mind and a part of our lives. By spending a little time out of the day to be mindful and contemplate our relationship with IF, we further our confidence and can develop a firm grasp of our goals and aspirations. Maintaining awareness of our body and mind is important to our goals in this book and an important practice to implement every day because our mindset and perception of a situation affect us subtly.

We emphasize awareness and mindfulness so much in this book for a good reason. We see the ancient cultures using fasting with great success, and their practices in mindfulness and awareness are certainly key to this success. Old practices like meditation and deep thought were very important to overall wellbeing in ancient philosophy. And so, as we see our ancestors and their practices permeating our current world, being studied in scientific settings and utilized in everyday life, we must give credit where credit is due and acknowledge that these practices are a very important aspect of existence. While keeping this in mind, let's move forward. Here, we begin the physical journey. We need to choose what type of fast works for us, schedule our meals, and then begin.

First things first, how do you want to fast? Choosing a practice type will be tough at first, and more often than not, the first course of action is not the one we stick with. You can do a little customization there, and some slight changes here. It is your practice, so do what you feel is best for you and not what everyone else is doing. We cannot tell you everything to do, but here are some helpful tips for the weeks leading up to the first fast:

- Think about it. Think of yourself and what you want to accomplish. Consider your food consumption and how it affects your body and mind. Prepare mentally for challenges that you will face – hunger, physical changes, emotions, and other drastic changes – that accompany this practice.

- Prepare physically. If you find that you're are in poor health, you may want to start changing little things in the week or two leading up to the fast. Cut back on desserts and detrimental foods, take a walk and other casual exercises, or chat with friends and family about what you're trying to accomplish to find support.

- Meal prep. Many people find that organizing meals beforehand helps them be on track. Buying reusable containers and preparing a week's worth of meals to keep in the fridge helps save time and ensures you keep your diet right for the fast.

- Ease in. Many feel that jumping right into a fast is shocking to their bodies, so the week before your major fast, maybe do half of what you planned for the big week. Maybe pick a fasting technique and use it for one or two days.

By preparing yourself beforehand, there's less of a chance that you will fail or have to restart the fast. You will be ready for any changes or unexpected outcomes that may find their way to you. Do not be disheartened if you cannot complete a fast the first time around. Everyone is different, and some people take the calorie restriction easier than others. If you have issues getting started, do not give up. Change your plan as you see fit; even if you only make it twenty-five percent of the week, you still have begun your transformation; you have still started changing your life for the better. The subtlest of changes have begun as soon as you started thinking about changing yourself. Be confident in yourself and your convictions. It's quite all right to fail; this is where we learn the most about ourselves. In fact, failing can even be viewed as an exercise in mindfulness. You learn from your mistakes and can try a different approach the next time around.

All in all, do not give up. If you truly value yourself and your life, this should be plenty of motivation to continue onward until you reach your goals. Having prepared yourself mentally and physically, success is inevitable.

Once we have given our schedule, lifestyle, and personal needs some thorough thought, we need to think even deeper about our personal goals. Are you seeking simply to lose a few pounds? Are you only curious about IF and not sure about the beginning? How will starting a fasting routine affect your lifestyle and the people around you? The questions are infinite in this context, but for all our intents and purposes with this book, we have a loose set of goals that we aim to achieve:

- Ridding ourselves of excess fat

- Developing a mindful and aware perception of health

- Adjusting our diets to suit a healthful lifestyle

- Maintaining any progress, we achieve (keep weight off, maintain awareness)

Through the combination of the goals above, we'll transform our lives for the better.

This list is presented as a general and vague overview of our intentions with this book. Even if you only want to lose a few pounds, doing so will also transform your mindset and awareness, whether it's intentional or not. Develop a personal list with the above goals in mind. The list can be anything you want to change: weight loss, health, new job, new home, etc. Anything you desire, add it to this list and think about how a healthier lifestyle can affect these things. From the mundane to the most important, feel free to be as specific as you need to be with your goals. You can apply these lifestyle changes to other aspects of your life too. Improving your health will inevitably touch all corners of your life, so setting goals outside the scope of physical health is quite all right. As we move forward, let's also take time to visualize ourselves as the people we wish to be. Visualize yourself at peak performance, visualize your life and surroundings as you truly want to be. This image will act as motivation and also as a primer for your mindfulness practice. The body and mind work together as one, so treat them as equals as we embark on our newfound Intermittent Fasting lifestyle.

Intermittent Fasting Rules

Settle for the Right Eating Window

Before determining when you will be fasting, it is worthwhile that you consider your everyday schedule. You cannot choose a feeding window period because your friend thinks it is best for you. It is vital that you mull over your demands. How much weight are you expecting to lose in 2-3 months? If you have set high goals, then you should go for a stricter fasting strategy. On the other hand, if you wish to take the fasting processes slowly, you can start slowly as you progress.

Think about the habits that you find difficult to change. This could be eating breakfast or dinner with your family. Maybe this is something that you have done for years. In such a scenario, you should settle for a window period that allows you to spend time with your family as you have been used to. This could mean that an ideal fasting period for you will be 12 hours during the day. Hence, eating breakfast early and a late dinner will work fine. The important thing that you should reflect on is a technique that suits you.

Drink Plenty of Water

Whether you are starting to fast or you have been doing this for a while, water will help you forget that you are hungry. Besides drinking water, you can opt to take in unsweetened coffee or tea. Don't add sugar to your drinks, as this will have an impact on your ketosis.

Exercise When You Have Energy

Some people will want to hasten their weight loss process by exercising regularly. It should be noted that this might be affected by your fasting window. Consequently, you should always listen to your body. If you feel tired, the best thing to do would be to rest. On the contrary, if you have enough energy at your disposal, burn those calories down.

Stay Busy

A huge challenge that most people face when fasting is that they find it awkward that they are staying away from food during breakfast, lunch, or dinner. For you to attain your weight loss goals, you should stay busy. This leaves your mind preoccupied and with little room to think about food.

Consistency is Key

Sure, consistency is difficult to achieve. Often, you will be tempted to eat. Expect this to happen so that you don't end up feeling frustrated. Admit that it's okay to slip from time to time. Nevertheless, you should not give up. Maintaining your consistency will ensure that your body adapts to your new eating habits.

Importance of Intermittent Fasting

Intermittent fasting can boost health in many ways if done appropriately. Various research studies prove that IF affects human wellbeing positively.

Effects on Hormones and Cells

Fasting affects the cellular and molecular processes of your body. Your body produces hormones to burn the stored fat for producing energy when you are not eating for more extended periods.

The human growth hormone or HGH increases during intermittent fasting up to five times. This increase in HGH promotes muscle gain and fat loss.

As mentioned earlier, insulin levels decrease during the fasted state. Consequently, the stored fat in the body is consumed to run the system.

Our body produces free radicals, which damage the vital body cells like DNA and protein. This process leads to aging and many chronic diseases. Intermittent fasting enhances the resistance against oxidative stress, according to many health studies. Mostly, oxidative stress occurs when there are many toxins accumulated in your body. Intermittent fasting detoxes your body by burning excessive fat and bad cells.

The cells also start repairing the damages and modify the gene expression. This repairing process is called autophagy. During autophagy, cells eliminate the wastage, including dysfunctional and old proteins gathered inside the cells. The genes' expressions are modified about immunity and longevity. These variations lead to better internal processes and a reduced aging process.

Intermittent fasting turbocharges your cells in many ways. It improves the regenerative capabilities of stem cells. On the other hand, it reduces the destruction of mitochondria too. Mitochondria are called the powerhouse of your body cells. If they are healthy, your body will be automatically healthy.

Simplifying the routine

You don't have to worry about your breakfast and, in some cases, about lunch as well, when fasting. Moreover, you don't have to count calories if you want to lose weight because you have restricted time for eating. So, no more stress about what to eat makes life easier, along with saving your cooking time.

Increasing lifespan

Controlling calorie intake is a proven way to prolong the lifespan. Intermittent fasting triggers several processes that slow down the wear and tear in your body. As a result, the aging process slows down.

Reducing the Risk of Cancer

Intermittent fasting detoxifies the body by burning the extra and damaged cells. Cancer is a disease of unwanted growth of cells in the body. Controlled eating during intermittent fasting decreases the growth of these harmful cells in your body. The process of detoxification and restricted growth of cells can reduce the risk of cancer to some extent.

The Easiest Diet Plan

Most people cannot follow a diet plan for a long time. This happens because almost every diet allows only a few food types, which become boring a few days after starting. For example, in the ketogenic diet, you cannot eat carbohydrates or sugar. This means no bread, pasta, pizza, and sweets.

Moreover, our body needs all the food groups to work correctly. Intermittent fasting allows you to eat whatever you want but within a restricted time. This is an inclusive diet schedule, and you can prepare your meals according to your taste.

Lower Stress Level

In typical dieting, keeping a strict check on calorie intake, eliminating your favorite foods from the diet, hunger pangs, and the feeling of deprivation causes stress and depression. This depression again results in excessive eating, which ruins all the effort done to control the weight. You can enjoy your favorite sweet dish, snack, or comfort food with carbohydrates any time before you start the fast again.

The flexibility that intermittent fasting allows compared to the other restricted diet plans gives you a sense of freedom and autonomy. The only thing you take care of is the duration of your eating. The motivation level of the people practicing intermittent fasting is found high during a study in comparison to those following other diet plans.

Weight loss

Dieting for weight loss has become a cliché nowadays. Most people start dieting because they want to lose weight. You consume fewer meals, which automatically reduces the calorie intake. Moreover, you have to quit eating after a certain period until you break your fast. This practice again restricts the amount of food you eat. Consequently, your body has to burn the already stored fat, which results in weight loss.

Along with that, as mentioned above, intermittent fasting activates the hormones promoting weight loss. Additionally, decreasing insulin level in the blood intensifies the release of norepinephrine, a fat-burning hormone. This hormone may increase the metabolic rate from three to fourteen times.

A study conducted in 2014 found that intermittent fasting can root three to eight percent weight loss within a period of three to twenty weeks. This change is noteworthy as compared to the other diet plans. The same study concluded that people who lost weight through intermittent fasting reduced their waist circumference as well. This reduction in their waist measurement means they lost their belly fat also, which is considered the most stubborn fat to cut. This fat doesn't only look bad but also causes diseases of the vital organs. This way, intermittent fasting can reduce the risk of potential heart, lungs, and stomach and kidney diseases.

Weight loss is not only about looking beautiful and fit, but it protects you from many diseases as well. Heart issues, joint pains, and diabetes are some diseases that you can get if you are overweight. Intermittent fasting helps you to reduce the risk of such diseases by healthily reducing your weight.

According to another research, you lose lesser muscle mass during intermittent fasting than any other way of a calorie-restricted diet.

All these factors boost the weight loss process and make intermittent fasting one of the best weight-loss strategies. But if you manage to eat more of calories and more substantial meals even during intermittent fasting, you may gain weight instead of losing any of your accumulated body fat.

Reduced risk of type 2 diabetes

Due to the lower release of insulin in the blood, there are fewer chances of you having type 2 diabetes when you are fasting.

Intermittent fasting can lower blood sugar levels by up to six percent and insulin level by thirty percent. These facts and figures must lead to the protection and control of type 2 diabetes. So, if you have a history of diabetes in your family or are diagnosed as a pre-diabetes patient, intermittent fasting can help you stay healthy.

The weight you lose as a result of intermittent fasting makes you insulin sensitive and keeps the blood sugar level down.

Inflammation

Your body loses damaged cells and waste during intermittent fasting, and this way reduces inflammation. Inflammation is mostly caused by the toxic materials gathered in the human body, and it may lead to severe and chronic health issues. Inflammation of soft tissues includes liver, intestines, kidneys, and lungs inflammation, which may be fatal. By removing toxins from your body and reducing inflammation, intermittent fasting helps you stay safe from the potential risk of such ailments.

Improved heart health

Increased levels of LDL or bad cholesterol, blood triglycerides, and inflammation are the risk factors for heart disease. Excessive body weight is also interlinked with heart problems, which can be effectively controlled by intermittent fasting.

Increased Brain health

The brain hormone BDNF increases as a result of intermittent fasting. This hormone is responsible for the growth of nerve cells. This way, all the brain diseases which are caused by the slow growth of new brain cells can be overcome. Alzheimer's disease is a chronic brain problem that gradually leads to memory loss and loss of coordination in the movement of various body parts. The scientists still have not discovered any effective treatment for it. The only way to stay safe is to protect against it. This new growth of brain cells boosted by intermittent fasting can prevent you from having Alzheimer's disease.

As intermittent fasting reduces inflammation of the soft tissues, it affects the brain as well. So, the local conditions of swelling of the brain and the problems caused by them can be controlled to some extent through intermittent fasting.

Parkinson's disease is also a dangerous brain condition that develops slowly and cannot be cured. Like Alzheimer's disease, the only way to protect against it is to promote new brain cells' growth. Intermittent fast protects you from Parkinson's disease by helping in the growth of healthy nerve cells.

Different types of IF

Before going further, you should keep in mind that you should try to keep your food intake as low as possible and avoid junk foods or highly processed foods during your eating period.

Following the ketogenic diet will take care of that, so no worries!

That being said, here are the different types of IF regimens.

The 16/8 method: This method is adjusted so that you fast for 14-16 hours per day, which gives you an eating window of 8-10 hours per day.

Within that eating time, you are allowed to go for 2-3 meals of your choice.

For example, if you finish your last meal at about 8:00 pm, you cannot eat until noon the next day. That's it!

Keep in mind, though, that you can consume coffee, water, and other zero-calorie beverages during the fasting period.

Eat-Stop-Eat protocol: This involves a 24-hour fast once or twice per week. A fitness expert, Brad Pilon, popularized this.

You are required to fast from the dinner of one day to the dinner of the next (24 hours).

You can also go for breakfast-to-breakfast or lunch-to-lunch if you prefer.

For example, you can have dinner at 7:00 pm on Monday and have your next meal on Tuesday at 7:00 pm.

Since the fast goes for 24 hours, it might be difficult for some people to follow this, so be sure to assess your limits before deciding on following this properly.

Alternate-day method: This form of fasting will ask you to fast every other day.

There are multiple variations of this fast depending on your requirements, but as a general rule of thumb, you are to keep your calories under 500 on fasting days.

However, since you are fasting for a whole day, this would be rather extreme for beginners, and I personally don't recommend it to newcomers.

The warrior diet: This particular diet was popularized by yet another expert known as Ori Hofmekler, and it involves eating very small amounts of raw veggies and fruits during the day, followed by a heavy meal at night.

Generally speaking, you fast throughout the day and feast for 4 hours at night.

Clean eating and paleo recipes are highly suitable for this form of fasting.

Spontaneous meal skip: This regimen won't give you a strict time frame as to when you are to skip your meals; rather, it gives you the option to personalize your fasting options and skip meals from time to time, depending on your level of comfort.

If you are not feeling hungry, then you may skip breakfast and follow it up with a healthy dinner, perhaps.

Skipping 1 or 2 meals every day is known as spontaneous intermittent fasting and is a very natural and accessible method for newcomers.

Why Do Both? The Benefits of Combined Keto Diet and Intermittent Fasting

The perfect diet to go with intermittent fasting is the ketogenic diet, as they utilize the same physiological and biochemical process, both ending up in regulated weight loss. Though they were from different areas of the weight loss method spectrum, they are in sync in terms of goals and methods. They both have a synergistic effect on one another.

For one, intermittent fasting utilizes ketones too because, in the state of starvation, your body has no choice but to use ketones as sources of energy. This being said, intermittent fasting practitioners who are not feeding on the ketogenic diet are unvaryingly undergoing ketogenesis at some point. Constantly feeding on a high-fat, very-low-carb diet would amplify the effect of intermittent fasting by providing the much-needed dietary lipids for ketogenesis, thus efficiently utilizing ketones whilst undergoing fasting.

Next is the increase in the renewal of cells brought about by fasting. The old unproductive cells that add mass to the person are taken in by the body, therefore, helping people lose unwanted weight. Ketogenesis further improves this process by efficiently providing ketones for energy and allotting enough resources for the body to develop new and healthy cells. Obese and overweight people will benefit the most from this because of the increase in worn-out cells' consumption, thus alleviating the person from the extra weight he has.

Also, what we are teaching to the body here is to induce ketogenesis with calories present. This is the purpose of intermittent fasting. We alternate the fasting and feeding periods (as opposed to continuous fasting), thus training the body to induce ketogenesis even when feeding, thus sparing the person from unregulated hunger pangs and energy gap while still on his way to achieving his weight goal.

As a concrete example, let's say that your day 1 is of keto diet with high fat, very low carb, and moderate protein. We encourage the digestive and metabolic system to generate lots of ketones as a primer for intermittent fasting to jumpstart the process. Your day 2 should already include intermittent fasting, which would utilize the dietary fat intake you had yesterday. At some point within the duration of the actual fast, no dietary fat is present and, therefore, would utilize body fat, significantly helping in weight loss.

With ample discipline, the combination of intermittent fasting and the ketogenic diet is the attainable strategy for your weight loss journey. These weight loss protocols are surprisingly in sync with each other in terms of both bodily processes to overall weight loss mechanisms. These both synergistically increase the weight loss potential of the other and must be done strategically together.

Chapter 3: Intermittent Fasting and Keto: Potential Benefits of Practicing Both

The quickest way for the body to enter ketosis is through fasting. You should remember that intermittent fasting is not a diet like a keto. It is a strategy that helps you determine when to eat.

Now, before bringing fasting into your keto diet, you must understand why keto works well with intermittent fasting.

The idea of sticking to a keto diet and fasting makes a lot of sense. This is because the keto diet is composed of foods rich in fat. Therefore, it will be easy for you to fast without feeling hungry too soon.

So, why is it essential that you practice fasting while on a keto diet?

Advantages of Fasting on Keto

Enter into Ketosis Faster

Ketosis is a metabolic state reached by the body after producing ketones. During this state, the body relies on ketones and fat as its main source of fuel. Fasting is the quickest way to ensure that the body enters into this metabolic state. Consequently, one of the main reasons it is recommended that you fast on keto is that it makes it easier for the body to begin producing ketones. In other words, it would be relatively easier for the body to begin burning fats.

Lose Weight Faster

Intermittent fasting and ketosis work hand in hand simply because they help your body reach a common goal - to reduce weight. In ketosis, the body depends on fat as its source of fuel. Therefore, the burning of these fats in the body will help you cut weight fast. You will be consuming less through your fasting routine, which will mean that losing weight will not be as challenging.

The Advantage of Calorie Restriction

Keto diet and intermittent fasting will help you maintain the right nutrition that your body needs to lose weight. This means that you will have to cut down your calorie intake.

Boost Mental Clarity

The body, the better it is, the more ketones it produces. This is because the brain will have plenty of energy reserved for its optimal use. Ultimately, this leads to a huge boost in mental clarity.

Makes Dieting Simpler

You cannot ignore the fact that dieting will be easier when you combine intermittent fasting with the keto diet. Sure, it will be somewhat difficult for you to stick to a keto diet. However, since you will be fasting, you will not worry about what you have to eat. Hence, it makes it easy for you to diet.

General Health Improvement

There are numerous benefits that you will get by simply choosing to fast.

Fasting is associated with improved metabolism. Regular fasting will, therefore, help enhance your metabolic health. Besides this, your muscles will grow effectively. Your body will also gain from its enhanced insulin sensitivity bearing in mind that it will be taking a break from regular insulin intake.

Always remember that fasting is not enough for you to lose weight effectively. As such, your fasting ought to be combined with the right supply of nutrition. Moreover, during this period, you should aim to reduce stress by getting enough sleep.

At the onset of your fasting exercise, you might find it difficult to fast for long hours. To deal with this, start by trying to adapt to a keto diet. This will help your body to last longer without going hungry.

It will be easy to fast with time, and therefore, you will find it natural just to stay away from food for a prolonged period.

In a word, fasting while on a keto diet is highly recommended. You will not only lose weight fast, but you will also gain other health benefits, including reversing type 2 diabetes.

Chapter 4: Should You Combine Them?

Is It Safe to Combine Both?

Yes, as long as a carefully structured schedule and menu have been prepared, and no other comorbidities are involved, doing intermittent fasting and ketogenic diet together is relatively safe, as opposed to more extreme dietary and fasting restrictions. The physiological processes involved are all-natural adaptations of our bodies that our ancestors have utilized in times of lesser resources such as famines. This combination protocol aims to take advantage of the innate capacity of the body to use its own stored body fat for energy and thus achieve weight loss.

What should be noted is the period of fasting to have sufficient energy during periods of work still. This is true, especially for beginners who still are carbohydrate-dependent in energy and are still in the process of efficiently using ketones as an energy source. The time of fasting must be matched to the lowest activity period to prevent being sluggish during activities requiring energy. Be strategic in timing your fasting and meals to prevent this problem.

For people with diabetes mellitus, intermittent fasting must be monitored carefully due to unregulated insulin. It may result in diabetic ketoacidosis, a state where the blood is at a lower pH, thus becoming acidic and may disturb vital functions. The ketogenic diet, where fatty foods are encouraged, must be monitored by people with hypertension and atherosclerosis history. Other than this, a carefully structured ketogenic diet and intermittent fasting protocol are safe when followed well.

Intermittent fasting can help you achieve ketosis more rapidly than after practicing a ketogenic diet alone. This is feasible as the body gets its energy from fats instead of carbohydrates when you practice intermittent fasting, as well as the ketogenic diet. So if you discover it difficult to enter a ketosis state, it can greatly assist you.

Food quality is more important than the amount here. Ideal products include grass-fed meat, pasture-grown hens' eggs, grass-fed butter and cheese, fruit, organic creams, and vegetables. They are ideal, but eating standard foods won't prevent ketosis from occurring. Do what you can to consume food of high quality.

In the ketogenic diet, you should consume lots of fat as they are the main source of energy, which doesn't imply you can eat fat without a limit. There are some good fats for you and others that aren't. A lot of saturated fats from poultry, eggs, meat, coconut, and butter must be eaten: polyunsaturated fats such as tuna and salmon; and monounsaturated fats such as nuts, nut butter, avocado, and olive oil. It is important to avoid highly produced polyunsaturated fats such as vegetable oil and soybean oil.

It is possible to obtain protein from many sources of fat, such as meat and eggs. You can also consume protein and fat, bacon, and sausages. To maintain you in ketosis, you should consume within the suggested grams of protein, as your body transforms the surplus protein into glucose.

Since fruits contain sugar, however natural they may be, they will boost your blood glucose and pull you out of ketosis state. Fruits are not completely prohibited; it relies on your consumption amount. It is best to consume fruits elevated in fiber and low in carbohydrates. On the other side, vegetables are essential because they supply minerals and vitamins without adding a lot of calories. They are helping to keep you safe. Some vegetables are full of carbohydrates, so the ketogenic diet is not permitted for all vegetables. Eat vegetables such as spinach, broccoli and green beans, asparagus, cucumbers, and mushrooms, leafy or pale green. Keep away from starchy vegetables such as white potatoes, yams, maize, and sweet potatoes.

Full-fat dairy is common in a ketogenic diet. Use heavy cream, sour cream, hard cheese, butter, and cottage cheese to help you satisfy your fat requirements. Avoid dairy products that are low-fat and flavored as they are full of sugar.

Water is the finest drink you can consume. You should always try to drink in ounces about half of your body weight. Unsweetened tea and coffee are permitted. Keep away from sodas, flavored water, and sweetened lemonade.

Grain and sugar consumption should be prevented in all types. Grains are like rice, rye, wheat, sorghum, barley, and any of its products. This means no pasta, no bread, and no crackers. It is not permitted to use honey, brown and white sugar, maple syrup, and anything else that includes sugar. Make sure there is no sugar in what you consume.

The combination of the two can lead to fat melting quicker than each on its own. During intermittent fasting, your body utilizes stubborn fat as it encourages metabolism that results in heat manufacture. This helps preserve muscle mass during weight loss and increases energy levels for keto dieters who want to lose weight and improve their athletic prowess. Combining the scheme of intermittent fasting drinking and the calorie counting and drinking regimen of the ketogenic diet can lead to more body fat melting than individuals who still consume junk food.

It can also increase your body structure as intermittent fasting improves the human growth hormone output but a very large proportion. This hormone performs an enormous part in constructing muscles. According to studies conducted, the human growth hormone helps an individual reduce body fat concentrations and boost lean body and bone mass. Working out in a fasted state can result in metabolic adjustments in your muscle cells arising in energy fat burning. The human growth hormone also enables you to recover from injury or even difficult exercise at a quicker pace. It also decreases skin swelling. It enhances the strength of your skin to wrinkles and sagging.

The mixture of the two can even affect the aging process in a beneficial way. They cause the manufacturing of stem cells to rise. These are like construction blocks for the body as they can be transformed into any cell the body requires and replace ancient or harmed cells, which keeps you younger internally for longer. These stem cells can do wonders for old wounds, chronic pain, and much more. This can enhance your life expectancy as your general health is enhanced by balancing blood glucose, reducing swelling, and improving the free radical defense.

It can boost autophagy. This is simply cell cleaning measures. When it starts, your cells migrate through your inner components and remove any harmed or old cells and replace them with fresh ones. It's like an organ upgrade. It decreases inflammation and improves organ life.

There are no cravings, tiredness, and mood changes when exercising the ketogenic diet and intermittent fasting. This is accomplished through constantly small concentrations of blood sugar. This is because your blood sugar concentrations are not increased by fat. You will be prepared to keep small blood sugar concentrations that can significantly assist individuals with form 2 diabetes, even get off their drugs.

The liver transforms fat into packets of energy called ketones that are taken into the blood to offer your cells energy. These ketones destroy ghrelin, the primary hunger hormone. High concentrations of ghrelin leave you famished, while ketones decrease hormone concentrations, even if your digestive tract does not contain any meals. This means you can stay without eating for a longer time and won't get hungry. Undoubtedly, the ketogenic diet makes fasting much easier for you to do.

Some individuals have the ketogenic diet integrated with intermittent fasting. This is by observing the ketogenic nutritional laws while also pursuing the trend of intermittent fasting eating. This can have many advantages, including high-fat burning levels, as both are important in using fats for energy over carbohydrates, providing you energy, reducing cholesterol in your body, controlling your blood sugar that can assist manage type 2 diabetes, helping to cope with hunger, and reducing skin inflammation.

Combining the two is comfortable for most individuals and can significantly speed up the fat burning process, making you accomplish your objectives quicker. However, one or the other can be done alone as they have many comparable advantages. Choosing an intermittent fasting unit that fits you is also essential, and always makes sure you consume enough of the macro ingredients. Depending on what was in the meals, the functions can be comparatively fine for both. The job performed will be ideal when you mix both of them and will make weight loss much easier for you to do as both operate in distinct aspects but complement each other superbly.

PART TWO: MEAL PLAN AND RECIPES

Chapter 5: Keto and IF 21-days Meal Plan

Shopping List-What to buy and what not to buy

Fats Go for...

Saturated fat like coconut oil or ghee

Monosaturated fat like olive, macadamia, and almond oils

Polyunsaturated Omega 3s as sardines

Medium-chain triglycerides such as fatty acid

Lard

Chicken fat

Duck fat

Goose fat

Do not go for...

Refined fats and oils such as sunflower, soybean, corn oil, etc.

Trans fat such as margarine

Protein Go for...

Grass-fed meat

Harvested seafood and wild-caught meat

Free-range organic eggs

Beef

Lamb

Goat

Venison

Pastured pork

Poultry

Do not go for...

Factory-packed animal foods and products

Vegetables Go for...

Leafy green vegetables

Low-carb vegetables

Swiss chard

Bok choy

Lettuce

Chard

Chives

Endive

Radicchio

Do not go for...

High-starch, high-carb vegetables such as peas, potatoes, yucca, and legumes

Dairy Products Go for...

Dairy products such as yogurt, sour cream, cottage cheese, goat cheese, and whole milk

Do not go for...

Low-fat or skim milk, etc.

Fruits Go for...

In general, go for fruits that are low on carbs and/or have more fat, such as berries, avocados, etc.

Do not go for...

Try to avoid dried fruits that are high in sugar content

Drinks Go For...

Water

Black Coffee

Unsweetened and Herbal Teas

Nut Milk

Light Beet

Wine

Do not go for...

Drinks such as Pepsi or Coke

High Fructose Syrup

Nectar

Honey

Sodas

Sweets Go For...

Stevia

Xylitol

Erythritol

Inulin

Monk Fruit Powder

Cocoa Dark Chocolate

Meal Plan

DAY	BREAKFAST	LUNCH/DINNER	SNACK/DESSERT
1	Cheese Crepes	Sausage and Pepper Soup	Keto Bulletproof Coffee
2	Blueberry Pancakes	Hearty Shrimp Curry	Almond Butter Bulletproof Coffee
3	Savory Broccoli Muffins	Ancient Salmon Glaze and Teriyaki	Raspberry Chia Pudding
4	Flax Seeds Bread	Extremely Low Carb Chicken Satay	Raspberry Chocolate Fudge
5	Pumpkin Bread	Spicy Hot Chicken and Pepper Soup	Strawberry Chia Pudding Popsicles
6	Cheddar Scramble	Butter Fried Kale and Pork With Cranberries	Almond Butter Cookies

7	Bacon & Cheddar Omelet	Amazing Keto Zucchini Hash	Caramelized Onions
8	Chicken & Asparagus Frittata	Steak and Broccoli Stir Fry	Curry Mayonnaise
9	Chocolate Smoothie	Salmon and Green Beans	Green Tahini
10	Vanilla Smoothie	Stuffed Zucchini	Cheesy Fondue
11	Strawberry Cow Smoothie	Creamy Zucchini Noodles	Green Bean Fries
12	Golden Milk Smoothie	Cauliflower Crust Pizza	Seed Crackers & Guacamole
13	Almond Butter Smoothie	Cabbage Casserole	Celery and Almond Butter

14	Pink Power Smoothie	Salmon with Salsa	
15	Cheese Crepes	Salmon & Veggie Parcel	Salted Macadamias
16	Blueberry Pancakes Savory Broccoli Muffins	Bacon & Jalapeño Soup	Nordic Seed Bread
17	Flax Seeds Bread	Broccoli Soup	Almond Butter Fat Bombs
18	Pumpkin Bread	Yellow Squash Soup	Mediterranean Fat Bombs
19	Cheddar Scramble	Chicken Soup	Keto Bulletproof Coffee

20	Bacon & Cheddar Omelet	Meatballs Soup	Almond Butter Bulletproof Coffee
21	Chicken & Asparagus Frittata	Broiled Tilapia Creamy & Cheesy Steak	Raspberry Chia Pudding

Chapter 6: Recipes

Breakfast Recipes

Cheese Crepes

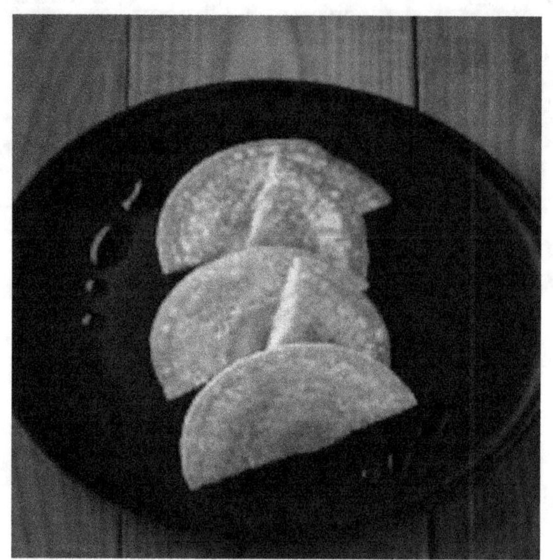

Servings: 2

Preparation time: 15 minutes

Cooking time: 20 minutes

Allergens: egg, dairy

Ingredients:

6 ounces of cream cheese, softened

1/3 cup of Parmesan cheese, grated

6 large organic eggs

1 teaspoon of Erythritol

1½ tablespoons of coconut flour

1/8 teaspoon of xanthan gum

2 tablespoons of unsalted butter

Directions

In a blender, add the cream cheese, Parmesan cheese, eggs, and Erythritol and pulse on low speed until well combined.

While the motor is running, place the coconut flour and xanthan gum and pulse until a thick mixture is formed.

Now, pulse on medium speed for about 5-10 seconds.

Transfer the mixture into a bowl and set aside for at least 5 minutes.

In a nonstick frying pan, melt the butter over medium-low heat.

Add ¼ cup of the mixture and tilt the pan to spread into a thin layer.

Cook for about 1½ minutes or until the edges become brown.

Carefully flip the crepe and cook for about 15-20 seconds more.

Repeat with the remaining mixture.

Serve warm with your favorite keto-friendly filling.

Nutrition: Calories: 283

Fat: 24.3g Sat Fat: 13.5g Cholesterol: 200mg Sodium: 274mg Carbohydrates: 3.8g Fiber: 1.6g Sugar: 0.8g Protein: 12.9g

Blueberry Pancakes

Servings: 2

Preparation time: 15 minutes

Cooking time: 21 minutes

Allergens: egg, nuts

Ingredients:

½ cup of almond flour

2 tablespoons of coconut flour

½ teaspoon of organic baking powder

1 teaspoon of ground cinnamon

1½ tablespoons of Erythritol

¼ cup of unsweetened almond milk

3 large organic eggs

¼ cup of fresh blueberries

Directions

In a high-speed blender, add all ingredients and pulse until a thick mixture is formed.

Place the mixture into a bowl and gently fold in blueberries.

Set aside for about 5-10 minutes.

Heat a lightly greased skillet over medium-low heat.

Add about ¼ cup of the mixture, and with the back of a spatula, spread it into desired thickness.

Immediately, cover the skillet and cook for about 4 minutes.

Uncover and carefully flip the side.

Cook for 3 minutes or until it turns golden brown.

Repeat with the remaining mixture.

Serve warm.

Nutrition: Calories: 231

Fat: 12.7g Sat Fat: 3.6g Cholesterol: 186mg Sodium: 106mg Carbohydrates: 12g Fiber: 6.1g Sugar: 2.9g Protein: 11.8g

Savory Broccoli Muffins

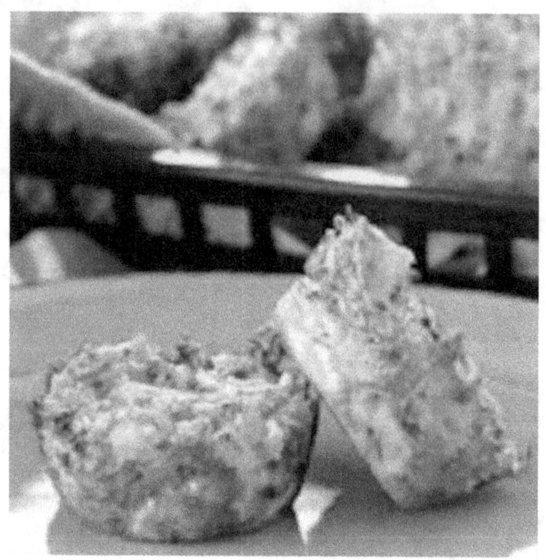

Servings: 2

Preparation time: 15 minutes

Cooking time: 20 minutes

Allergens: egg, dairy

Ingredients:

2 tablespoons of unsalted butter

6 large organic eggs

½ cup of heavy whipping cream

½ cup of Parmesan cheese, grated

Salt and ground black pepper, as required

1¼ cups of broccoli, chopped

2 tablespoons of fresh parsley, chopped

½ cup of Swiss cheese, grated

Directions

Preheat your oven to 350 F (180 C). Grease 12 cups of a muffin tin.

In a bowl, add the eggs, cream, Parmesan cheese, salt, and black pepper and beat until well mixed.

Divide the broccoli and parsley in the bottom of each prepared muffin cup evenly.

Top with the egg mixture, followed by the Swiss cheese.

Bake for about 20 minutes, rotating the pan once halfway through.

Remove from the oven and place onto a wire rack for about 5 minutes before serving.

Carefully invert the muffins onto a serving platter and serve warm.

Nutrition: Calories: 103

Fat: 8.3g Sat Fat: 4.4g Cholesterol: 112mg Sodium: 103mg Carbohydrates: 1.2g Fiber: 0.3g Sugar: 0.4g Protein: 6.1g

Flax Seeds Bread

Servings: 2

Preparation time: 15 minutes

Cooking time: 28 minutes

Allergens: egg, dairy

Ingredients:

2 cups of flax seeds meal

2 tablespoons of Swerve

1 tablespoon of organic baking powder

½ teaspoon of salt

5 organic eggs, beaten

5 tablespoons of unsalted butter, melted

½ cup of water

1 teaspoon of organic vanilla extract

Directions

Preheat your oven to 350 F (180 C). Line a 15x10-inch loaf pan with lightly greased parchment paper.

In a bowl, add the flax seeds meal, Swerve, baking powder, and salt, and mix.

In another bowl, add the eggs, butter, water, and vanilla extract and beat until well combined.

Add the egg mixture into the bowl with flax seeds meal mixture and mix until well combined.

Place the mixture into a prepared loaf pan.

Bake for about 24-28 minutes or until a toothpick inserted in the center comes out clean.

Remove the bread pan from the oven and place it onto a wire rack to cool for about 10 minutes.

Now, place the bread onto the wire rack to cool before slicing.

With a sharp knife, cut the bread loaf into desired sized slices and serve.

Nutrition: Calories: 196

Fat: 14.6g Sat Fat: 4.5g Cholesterol: 81mg Sodium: 158mg Carbohydrates: 9g Fiber: 6.3g Sugar: 0.2g Protein: 7.7g

Pumpkin Bread

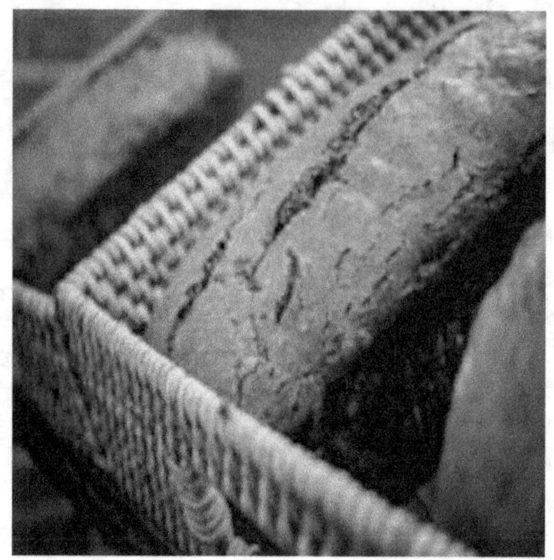

1 serving

Preparation time: 20 minutes

Cooking time: 1 hour

Allergens: egg, dairy, nuts

Ingredients:

1 2/3 cups of almond flour

1½ teaspoon of organic baking powder

½ teaspoon of pumpkin pie spice

½ teaspoon of ground cinnamon

½ teaspoon of ground cloves

½ teaspoon of salt

8 ounces of cream cheese, softened

6 organic egg, divided

1 tablespoon of coconut flour

1 cup of powdered Erythritol, divided

1 teaspoon of stevia extract powder, divided

1 teaspoon of lemon extract

1 cup of homemade pumpkin puree

½ cup of coconut oil, melted

Directions

Preheat your oven to 325 F (170 C). Lightly, grease 2 bread loaf pans.

In a bowl, add the almond flour, baking powder, spices, and salt, and mix until well combined.

In a second bowl, add the cream cheese, 1 egg, coconut flour, ¼ cup of Erythritol, and ¼ teaspoon of the stevia, and with a wire whisk, beat until smooth.

In a third bowl, add the pumpkin puree, oil, 5 eggs, ¾ cup of the Erythritol, and ¾ teaspoon of the stevia, and with a wire whisk, beat until well combined.

Add the pumpkin mixture into the bowl of the flour mixture and mix until it is well combined.

Place about ¼ of the pumpkin mixture into each loaf pan evenly.

Top each pan with the cream cheese mixture evenly, followed by the remaining pumpkin mixture.

Bake for about 50-60 minutes or until a toothpick inserted in the center comes out clean.

Remove the bread pan from the oven and place it onto a wire rack to cool for about 10 minutes.

Now, invert the bread onto the wire rack to cool before slicing.

With a sharp knife, cut each bread loaf into the desired sized slices and serve.

Nutrition: Calories: 208

Fat: 19.4g Sat Fat: 10.1g Cholesterol: 77mg Sodium: 142mg Carbohydrates: 5.1g Fiber: 2.1g Sugar: 1.1g Protein: 6g

Cheddar Scramble

Servings: 2

Preparation time: 10 minutes

Cooking time: 8 minutes

Allergens: egg, dairy

Ingredients:

2 tablespoons of olive oil

1 jalapeño pepper, chopped

1 small yellow onion, chopped

12 large organic eggs, beaten lightly

Salt and ground black pepper, as required

3 tablespoons of fresh chives, chopped finely

4 ounces of cheddar cheese, shredded

Directions

Heat oil in a large skillet over medium and sauté the jalapeño pepper and onion for about 4-5 minutes.

Add the eggs, salt, and black pepper and cook for about 3 minutes, stirring continuously.

Remove from the heat and immediately stir in the chives and cheese.

Serve immediately.

Nutrition: Calories: 265

Fat: 20.9g Sat Fat: 7.8g Cholesterol: 390mg Sodium: 285mg Carbohydrates: 2.3g Fiber: 0.4g Sugar: 1.5g Protein: 17.5g

Bacon & Cheddar Omelet

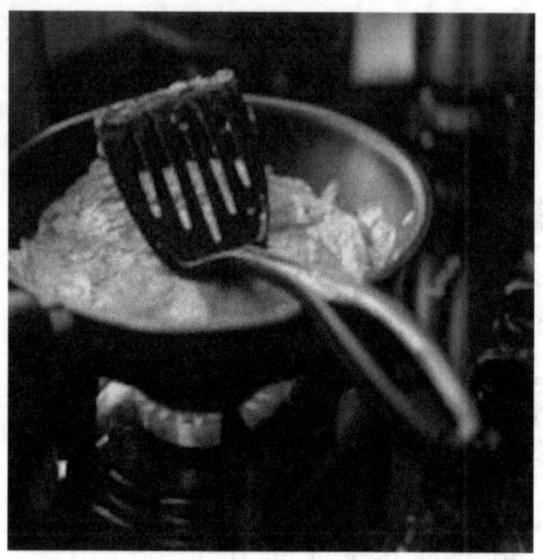

Servings: 2

Preparation time: 10 minutes

Cooking time: 15 minutes

Allergens: egg, dairy

Ingredients:

4 large organic eggs

1 tablespoon fresh chives, minced

Salt and ground black pepper, as required

4 bacon slices

1 tablespoon of unsalted butter

2 ounces of Cheddar cheese, shredded

Directions

In a bowl, add the eggs, chives, salt, and black pepper and beat until well combined.

Heat a nonstick frying pan over medium-high heat and cook the bacon slices for about 8-10 minutes.

Place the bacon onto a paper towel-lined plate to drain. Then chop the bacon slices.

With a paper towel, wipe out the frying pan.

In the same frying pan, melt the butter over medium-low heat and cook the egg mixture for about 2 minutes.

Carefully flip the omelet and top with chopped bacon.

Cook for 1-2 minutes or until the desired doneness of eggs.

Remove from heat and immediately place the cheese in the center of the omelet.

Fold the edges of the omelet over the cheese and cut it into 2 portions.

Serve immediately.

Nutrition: Calories: 633

Fat: 49.3g Sat Fat: 20.7g Cholesterol: 400mg Sodium: 1500mg Carbohydrates: 2g Fiber: 0g Sugar: 1g Protein: 41.2g

Chicken & Asparagus Frittata

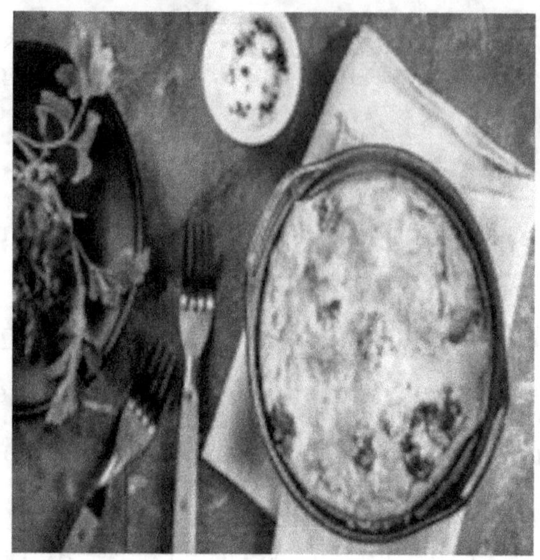

Servings: 2

Preparation time: 15 minutes

Cooking time: 12 minutes

Allergens: egg, dairy

Ingredients:

½ cup of grass-fed cooked chicken, chopped

1/3 cup of Parmesan cheese, grated

6 organic eggs, beaten lightly

Salt and ground black pepper, as required

1 teaspoon of unsalted butter

½ cup of boiled asparagus, chopped

1 tablespoon of fresh parsley, chopped

Directions

Preheat the broiler of the oven.

In a bowl, add the cheese, eggs, salt, and black pepper and beat until well combined.

In a large ovenproof skillet, melt butter over medium-high heat and cook the chicken and asparagus for about 2-3 minutes.

Add the egg mixture and stir to combine.

Cook for about 4-5 mins.

Remove from the heat and sprinkle with the parsley.

Now, transfer the skillet under broiler and broil for about 3-4 minutes or until slightly puffed.

Cut into desired sized wedges and serve immediately.

Nutrition: Calories: 157

Fat: 9.7g Sat Fat: 3.6g Cholesterol: 260mg Sodium: 207mg Carbohydrates: 1.2g Fiber: 0.4g Sugar: 0.8g Protein: 16.5g

Chocolate Smoothie

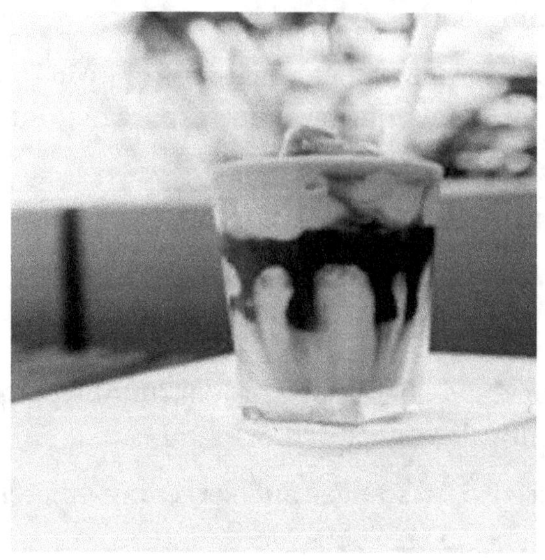

Servings: 1

Serving Size: whole recipe

Preparation Time: 5 minutes

Cooking Time: 0 minutes

Ingredients:

1 tablespoon of chia seeds

1 egg yolk

1 tablespoon of almond butter

1 tablespoon of cocoa butter

1/4 cup of heavy cream

1 tablespoon of cocoa powder

1 teaspoon of Stevia

1/2 cup of ice

1/4 teaspoon of chocolate essence (unsweetened) or 1/4 teaspoon of vanilla extract

Directions

Pour the ice and cream into the bottom of the blender to prevent the other ingredients from sticking to the bottom. Add in the rest of the ingredients and blend on high until smooth. Serve immediately.

Nutrition: 575 calories, 44 g fat, 34 g protein, 3 g net carbs

Vanilla Smoothie

Serving: 1

Serving Size: whole recipe

Preparation Time: 5 minutes

Cooking Time: 0 minutes

Ingredients

1 cup of coconut milk

1 tablespoon of coconut oil

1/2 tablespoon of vanilla extract

1 teaspoon of Stevia

Directions:

Combine all ingredients in a blender until smooth. Serve immediately.

Nutrition: 669 calories, 70.8g fat, 5.5 g protein, 4 g net carbs

Strawberry Cow Smoothie

Serving: 1

Serving Size: whole recipe

Preparation Time: 5 minutes

Cooking Time: 0 minutes

Ingredients

1/2 cup of frozen strawberries

1/2 cup of full fat coconut milk

1 cup of ice

Directions:

Pour the coconut milk into the bottom of the blender to prevent the other ingredients from sticking. Add in the rest of the ingredients and puree until smooth. Serve immediately.

Nutrition: 301 calories, 28.6 g fat, 2.8 g protein, 9 g net carbs

Golden Milk Smoothie

Serving: 1

Serving Size: whole recipe

Preparation Time: 5 minutes

Cooking Time: 0 minutes

Ingredients

1 tablespoon of turmeric

1 cup of coconut milk

1 teaspoon of Stevia

1 cup of crushed ice

Directions:

Puree all ingredients together until smooth. Serve immediately.

Nutrition: 460 calories, 25.3 g fat, 1.7g protein, 1.4 g net carbs

Almond Butter Smoothie

Serving: 2

Serving Size: about 1 cup

Preparation Time: 5 minutes

Cooking Time: 0 minutes

Ingredients

2 tablespoons of almond butter

1 1/2 cups of almond milk

1 tablespoon of hemp seeds

Directions:

Start by pouring the almond milk into the blender to avoid the ingredients sticking at the bottom. Add in the rest of the ingredients. Turn the blender on, starting at a low speed and increase as needed. Add extra water if you desire your smoothie more on the liquid side. Pour into a cup and serve immediately. Place any leftover smoothie into an airtight container and enjoy within 24 hours.

Nutrition: 483 calories, 34.6g fat, 5.5g protein, 4g net carbs

Pink Power Smoothie

Serving: 2

Serving Size: half recipe

Preparation Time: 5 minutes

Cooking Time: 0 minutes

Ingredients

1/2 cup of raspberries

1/2 tablespoon of lemon zest

1 cup of coconut milk

1 tablespoon of flaxseeds

Directions:

Start by pouring the coconut milk into the blender to avoid the ingredients sticking at the bottom. Add in the rest of the ingredients. Turn the blender on, start at a low speed and increase as needed. Add extra water if you desire your smoothie more on the liquid side. Once it looks even, pour it into a cup and serve immediately. Pour any leftover smoothie into an airtight container and enjoy within 24 hours.

Nutrition: 310 calories, 29.9g fat, 3.8g protein, 9g net carbs

Lunch Recipes

Sausage and Pepper Soup

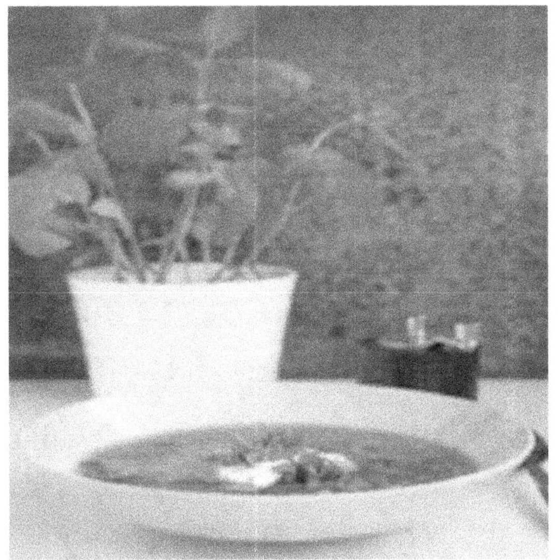

Servings: 2

Preparation Time: 10 minutes

Cooking Time: 45 minutes

Ingredients

32 ounces of Pork Sausages

1 tablespoon of Olive Oil

10 ounce of Raw Spinach

1 medium-sized Green Bell Pepper

1 can of jalapenos with tomatoes

4 cup of beef stock

1 tablespoon of chili powder

1 tablespoon of cumin

1 teaspoon of Garlic Powder

1 teaspoon of Italian Seasoning

¾ teaspoon of Salt

Directions

Take a large-sized pot and place it over medium heat

Add olive oil and allow the oil to heat up

Add sausages and cook until seared

Slice the green pepper into small pieces and add to the pot

Season with pepper and salt

Add tomatoes, jalapenos and give it a nice stir

Add spinach on top and cover with a lid

Once the spinach has wilted, add the remaining spices and beef stock

Cook on medium-low heat for 30 minutes more

Remove the lid and simmer for 15 minutes over low heat

Serve and enjoy!

Nutrition Values (Per Serving)

Protein: 27g

Carbs: 3.8g

Fats: 2.3g

Calories: 525

Hearty Shrimp Curry

Servings: 2

Preparation Time: 5 minutes

Cooking Time: 10 minutes

Ingredients

2 tablespoon of Green Curry paste

1 cup of vegetable stock

1 cup of coconut milk

6 ounce of Pre-Cooked shrimp

5 ounce of Broccoli florets

3 tablespoon of chopped cilantro

2 tablespoon of Coconut Oil

1 tablespoon of Soy Sauce

½ of a lime juice

1 medium-sized spring onion chopped up

1 teaspoon of crushed roasted garlic

1 teaspoon of minced garlic

1 teaspoon of fish sauce

½ teaspoon of Turmeric

¼ teaspoon of Xanthan Gum

½ of a cup of sour cream

Directions

Place a pan over medium heat and add two tablespoons of coconut oil

Add minced ginger, chopped up onion, and cook for a minute

Add turmeric and curry paste

Add a tablespoon of soy sauce, fish sauce, and mix

Add a cup of vegetable stock and a cup of coconut milk

Stir well and add green curry paste

Simmer

Add ¼ teaspoon of Xanthan Gum and mix well

After a while, you will notice that the curry will begin to thicken; that will be the moment when you are going to add the florets and stir them finely

Add the fresh chopped cilantro

Once you have a nice consistency, add weighed pre-cooked shrimp and lime juice

Allow the mix to simmer for a few minutes and season with pepper and salt

Serve with ¼ cup of sour cream

Enjoy!

Nutrition (Per Serving)

Protein: 27g

Carbs: 8.9g

Fats: 31g

Calories: 454

Ancient Salmon Glaze and Teriyaki

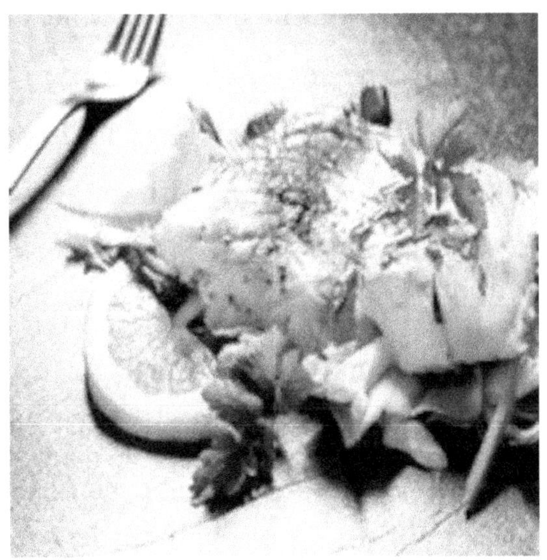

Servings: 2

Preparation Time: 10 minutes

Cooking Time: 10 minutes

Ingredients

10 ounces of Salmon Fillet

2 tablespoon of Soy Sauce

2 teaspoon of Sesame Oil

1 tablespoon of Rice Vinegar

1 teaspoon of Minced Ginger

2 teaspoon of Minced Garlic

1 tablespoon of Red Boat Fish Sauce

1 tablespoon of Sugar-Free Ketchup

2 tablespoon of Dry White Wine

Directions

Toss in all of the ingredients in a small-sized Tupperware. Just make sure not to toss the sesame oil, white wine, and ketchup

Marinade everything for about 10-15 minutes

Bring down the pan to a nice heat and toss in the sesame oil

Once the smoke is seen, toss the fish with the skin side down

Let it cook until crispy

Flip it and cook the other side

Each side should take about 3-4 minutes

Pour in the marinade liquid to the fish and let it boil

Slowly remove the fish from the pan and pour in the ketchup alongside the white wine to the liquid in the pan

Simmer for 5 minutes and serve as a side

Nutrition:

Protein: 33g

Carbs: 2.5g

Fats: 23.5g

Calories: 370

Extremely Low Carb Chicken Satay

Serving: 1

Preparation Time: 5 minutes

Cooking Time: 5 minutes

Ingredients

1 pound of Ground Chicken

4 tablespoon of Soy Sauce

2 onion springs

1/3 pieces of Yellow Pepper

1 tablespoon of Erythritol

1 tablespoon of Rice Vinegar

2 teaspoon of Sesame Oil

2 teaspoon of Chili Paste

1 teaspoon of Minced Garlic

1/3 teaspoon of Cayenne Pepper

¼ teaspoon of Paprika

Juice of ½ a lime

Directions

Add 2 teaspoon of sesame oil to a pan and heat it over medium-high heat

Add ground chicken to your pan and allow it to brown

Add the rest of the ingredients and mix well

Once the mixture has reached your desired texture, add 2 chopped up spring onion and 1/3 of your sliced yellow pepper

Mix and serve!

Nutrition:

Protein: 105g

Carbs: 18g

Fats: 69g

Calories: 1180

Spicy Hot Chicken and Pepper Soup

Servings: 2

Preparation Time: 5 minutes

Cooking Time: 10 minutes

Ingredients

1 teaspoon of Coriander Seeds

2 tablespoon of Olive Oil

2 sliced chili pepper

2 cups of chicken broth

2 cups of water

1 teaspoon of Turmeric

½ a teaspoon of Ground Cumin

4 tablespoon of Tomato Paste

16 ounce of chicken thigh

2 tablespoon of butter

1 medium-sized avocado

2 ounce of Queso Fresco

4 tablespoon of chopped cup Cilantro

Juice of a half lime

Salt as required

Pepper as required

Directions

Cut the chicken thigh into small portions

Take a pan and place it over medium heat, add oil and allow the oil to heat up

Add chicken pieces and brown them on both sides, transfer to a platter and keep it on the side

Add two tablespoon of olive oil to the pan and add coriander seeds, toast until nice fragrant starts to come out

Pour water, broth and simmer it over low heat

Season with pepper, turmeric, salt, ground cumin

Bring the mix to a simmer and add tomato paste, butter and stir well

Simmer for 10 minutes and add the juice

Add 4 ounce of cooked chicken thigh and mix well

Garnish with avocado, cilantro, and queso fresco

Enjoy!

Nutrition:

Protein: 28g

Carbs: 10.8g

Fats: 27g

Calories: 395

Butter Fried Kale and Pork with Cranberries

Servings: 2

Preparation Time: 10 minutes

Cooking Time: 10 minutes

Ingredients

3 ounces of butter

1 pound of kale

¾ pound of smoked pork belly

2 ounce of pecans

½ cup of frozen cranberries

Directions

Rinse, trim and chop your kale into large-sized chunks

Keep it on the side

Cut the pork belly into strips and fry them in butter over medium-high heat

Once they are golden brown and crispy, add kale to the pan and fry for a few minutes

Remove the heat and add cranberries and nuts to the pan

Stir well and serve!

Nutrition:

Protein: 21g

Carbs: 10g

Fats: 12g

Calories: 223

Amazing Keto Zucchini Hash

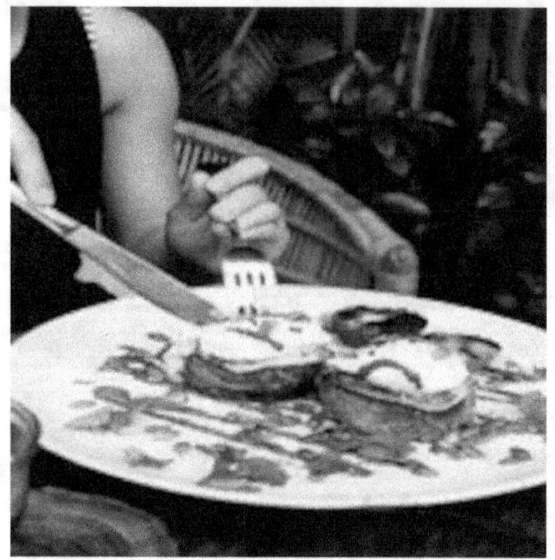

Servings: 2

Preparation Time: 10 minutes

Cooking Time: 10-15 minutes

Ingredients

1 medium-sized zucchini

2 slices of bacon

½ of a small white onion

1 tablespoon of coconut oil

1 tablespoon of freshly chopped parsley

¼ teaspoon of salt

1 large egg

Directions

Peel and finely chop up the onion and slice the bacon

Sweat the onions over medium heat and add the bacon; make sure to stir from time to time to ensure that they are lightly browned

Dice the zucchini into medium pieces

Add zucchini to your pan and cook for 10-15 minutes, remove from the heat and add chopped parsley

Top with a fried egg and enjoy!

Nutrition:

Protein: 17g

Carbs: 6g

Fats: 35g

Calories: 423

Steak and Broccoli Stir Fry

Serving: 2

Preparation Time: 10 minutes

Cooking Time: 10-15 minutes

Ingredients

4 ounce of butter

¾ pound of Ribeye steak

9 ounce of broccoli

1 yellow onion

1 tablespoon of tamari soy sauce

1 tablespoon of pumpkin seed

Salt as needed

Pepper as needed

Directions

Slice up the steak and onion

Slice/chop the broccoli, including the stems

Take a frying pan and place it over medium heat

Add butter and heat it, brown the meat

Season the meat with salt and pepper and keep it on the side

Brown the broccoli and onion in the same pan with a bit more butter

Save a dollop of butter for later

Add soy sauce towards the pan and return the meat to the pan, and stir

Season with some salt and pepper

Serve with a dollop of butter and sprinkle of pumpkin seeds

Nutrition:

Protein: 7g

Carbs: 9g

Fats: 15g

Calories: 196

Rotisserie Chicken and Cabbage Shreds

Servings: 2

Preparation Time: 5 minutes

Cooking Time: 0 minutes

Ingredients

1 pound of rotisserie chicken (cooked)

7 ounce of fresh green cabbage

½ of a red onion

1 tablespoon of olive oil

½ a cup of mayonnaise (Keto-Friendly recipe provided)

Salt as needed

Pepper as needed

Directions

Shred the cabbage using a sharp knife and place them on a plate

Slice the onion thinly and add them to the plate

Add rotisserie chicken to the plate

Add mayonnaise and drizzle with olive oil

Season with some pepper and salt and mix well

Enjoy!

Nutrition:

Protein: 17g

Carbs: 6g

Fats: 35g

Calories: 423

Salmon and Green Beans

Servings: 2

Preparation Time: 5 minutes

Cooking Time: 10 minutes

Ingredients

9 ounce of fresh green beans

3 and a ½ ounce of butter

9 ounce of salmon, cut up into small portions

Salt and pepper as needed

Directions

Rinse and trim your green beans

Take a frying pan and place it over medium-high heat

Add butter and melt it

Fry the green beans for 3-4 minutes, and season with salt and pepper

Place them on the side of the pan

Add a bit of butter and add the salmon pieces, fry them for a few minutes, making sure to keep stirring the beans from time to time

Lower down the heat

Season salmon and drizzle remaining butter

Serve and enjoy!

Nutrition:

Protein: 24g

Carbs: 12g

Fats: 22g

Calories: 349

Dinner Recipes

Stuffed Zucchini

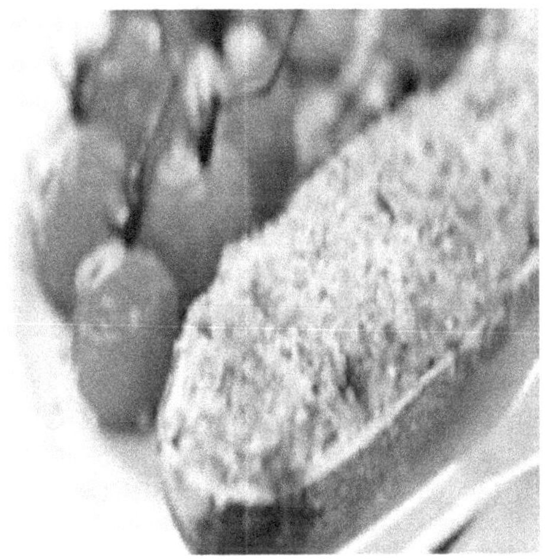

Servings: 2

Preparation time: 15 minutes

Cooking time: 18 minutes

Allergens: dairy

Ingredients:

4 medium zucchinis, halved lengthwise

1 cup of red bell pepper, seeded and minced

½ cup of Kalamata olives, pitted and minced

½ cup of fresh tomatoes, minced

1 teaspoon of garlic, minced

1 tablespoon of dried oregano, crushed

Salt and ground black pepper, as required

½ cup of feta cheese, crumbled

¼ cup of fresh parsley, chopped finely

Directions

Preheat your oven to 350 F (180 C). Grease a large baking sheet.

With a melon baller, scoop out the flesh of each zucchini half. Discard the flesh.

In a bowl, mix bell pepper, olives, tomato, garlic, oregano, and black pepper.

Stuff each zucchini half with the veggie mixture evenly.

Arrange the zucchini halves onto the prepared baking sheet and bake for about 15 minutes.

Now, set the oven to broiler on high.

Top each zucchini half with feta cheese and broil for about 3 minutes.

Garnish with parsley and serve hot.

Nutrition:

Calories: 60

Fat: 3.2g

Sat Fat: 1.6g

Cholesterol: 8mg

Sodium: 190mg

Carbohydrates: 6.4g

Fiber: 2g

Sugar: 3.2g

Protein: 3g

Creamy Zucchini Noodles

Servings: 2

Preparation time: 15 minutes

Cooking time: 10 minutes

Allergens: egg, dairy

Ingredients:

1¼ cups of heavy whipping cream

¼ cup of mayonnaise

Salt and ground black pepper, as required

30 ounces of zucchini, spiralized with blade C

4 organic egg yolks

3 ounces of Parmesan cheese, grated

2 tablespoons of fresh parsley, chopped

2 tablespoons of butter, melted

Directions

In a pan, add the heavy cream and boil.

Reduce the heat to low and cook until reduced.

Add the mayonnaise, salt, and black pepper, and cook until the mixture is warm enough.

Add the zucchini noodles and gently stir to combine.

Immediately, remove from the heat.

Place the zucchini noodles mixture onto 4 serving plates evenly and immediately, top with the egg yolks, followed by the parmesan and parsley.

Drizzle with butter and serve.

Nutrition:

Calories: 427

Fat: 39.1g

Sat Fat: 18.5g

Cholesterol: 297mg

Sodium: 412mg

Carbohydrates: 9.7g

Fiber: 2.4g

Sugar: 3.8g

Protein: 13g

Cauliflower Crust Pizza

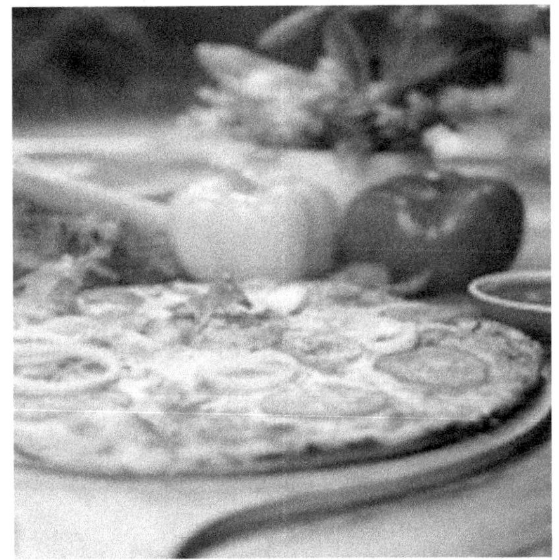

Servings: 2

Preparation time: 20 minutes

Cooking time: 42 minutes

Allergens: egg, dairy

Ingredients:

For Crust:

1 small head cauliflower, cut into florets

2 large organic eggs, beaten lightly

½ teaspoon of dried oregano

½ teaspoon of garlic powder

Ground black pepper, as required

For Topping:

½ cup of sugar-free pizza sauce

¾ cup of mozzarella cheese, shredded

¼ cup of black olives, pitted and sliced

2 tablespoons Parmesan cheese, grated

Directions

Preheat your oven to 400 F (200 C). Line a baking sheet with lightly greased parchment paper.

Add the cauliflower in a food processor and pulse until a rice-like texture is achieved.

In a bowl, add the cauliflower rice, eggs, oregano, garlic powder, and black pepper and mix until well combined.

Place the cauliflower the mixture in the center of the prepared baking sheet and, with a spatula, press into a 13-inch thin circle.

Bake for 40 minutes or until golden brown.

Remove the baking sheet from the oven.

Now, set the oven to broiler on high.

Place the tomato sauce on top of the pizza crust and, with a spatula, spread evenly and sprinkle with olives, followed by the cheeses.

Broil for about 1-2 minutes or until the cheese is bubbly and browned.

Remove from oven and with a pizza cutter, cut the pizza into equal-sized triangles.

Serve hot.

Nutrition:

Calories: 119

Fat: 6.6g

Sat Fat: 1.8g

Cholesterol: 98mg

Sodium: 297mg

Carbohydrates: 8.6g

Fiber: 3.4g

Sugar: 3.7g

Protein: 8.3g

Cabbage Casserole

Servings: 2

Preparation time: 15 minutes

Cooking time: 30 minutes

Allergens: dairy

Ingredients:

½ head cabbage

2 scallions, chopped

4 tablespoons of unsalted butter

2 ounces cream cheese, softened

¼ cup of Parmesan cheese, grated

¼ cup of fresh cream

½ teaspoon of Dijon mustard

2 tablespoons of fresh parsley, chopped

Salt and ground black pepper, as required

Directions

Preheat your oven to 350 F (180 C).

Cut the cabbage head into half, lengthwise. Then cut into 4 equal-sized wedges.

In a pan of boiling water, add cabbage wedges and cook, covered for about 5 minutes.

Drain well and arrange cabbage wedges into a small baking dish.

In a small pan, melt butter and sauté onions for about 5 minutes.

Add the remaining ingredients and stir to combine.

Remove from the heat and immediately place the cheese mixture over cabbage wedges evenly.

Bake for about 20 mins.

Remove from the oven and let it cool for about 5 minutes before serving.

Cut into 3 equal-sized portions and serve.

Nutrition:

Calories: 273

Fat: 24.8g

Sat Fat: 15.4g

Cholesterol: 71mg

Sodium: 313mg

Carbohydrates: 9g

Fiber: 3.4g

Sugar: 4.5g

Protein: 6.2g

Salmon with Salsa

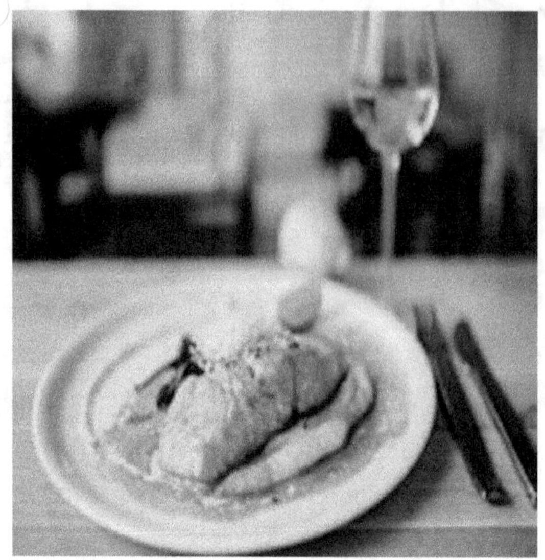

Servings: 2

Preparation time: 15 minutes

Cooking time: 8 minutes

Allergens: dairy

Ingredients:

For Salsa:

2 large ripe avocados, peeled, pitted, and cut into small chunks

1 small tomato, chopped

2 tablespoons of red onion, chopped finely

¼ cup of fresh cilantro, chopped finely

1 tablespoon of jalapeño pepper, seeded and minced finely

1 garlic clove, minced finely

3 tablespoons of fresh lime juice

Salt and ground black pepper, as required

For Salmon:

4 (5-ounce) (1-inch thick) salmon fillets

Sea salt and freshly ground black pepper, as required

3 tablespoons of butter

1 tablespoon of fresh rosemary leaves, chopped

1 tablespoon of fresh lemon juice

Directions

For the salsa: Add all ingredients in a bowl and gently stir to combine.

With plastic wrap, cover the bowl and refrigerate before serving.

For salmon: season each salmon fillet with salt and black pepper generously.

In a large skillet, melt butter over medium-high.

Place the salmon fillets, skins side up, and cook for about 4 minutes.

Carefully change the side of each salmon fillet and cook for about 4 minutes more.

Stir in the rosemary and lemon juice and remove from the heat.

Divide the salsa onto serving plates evenly.

Top each plate with 1 salmon fillet and serve.

Nutrition:

Calories: 481

Fat: 37.2g

Sat Fat: 10.9g

Cholesterol: 85mg

Sodium: 172mg

Carbohydrates: 11g

Fiber: 7.6g

Sugar: 1.5g

Protein: 29.9g

Salmon & Veggie Parcel

Servings: 2

Preparation time: 15 minutes

Cooking time: 20 minutes

Allergens: absent

Ingredients:

6 (3-ounce) salmon fillets

Salt and ground black pepper, as required

1 yellow bell pepper, seeded and cubed

1 red bell pepper, seeded and cubed

4 plum tomatoes, cubed

1 small yellow onion, sliced thinly

½ cup of fresh parsley, chopped

¼ cup of olive oil

2 tablespoons of fresh lemon juice

Directions

Preheat your oven to 400 F (200 C).

Arrange 6 pieces of foil onto a smooth surface.

Place 1 salmon fillet onto each foil paper and sprinkle with salt and black pepper.

In a bowl, add the bell peppers, tomato, and onion, and mix.

Place veggie mixture over each fillet evenly and top with parsley and capers.

Drizzle with oil and lemon juice.

Fold the foil around the salmon mixture to seal it.

Arrange the foil packets onto a large baking sheet in a single layer.

Bake for about 20 minutes.

Serve hot.

Nutrition:

Calories: 224

Fat: 14g

Sat Fat: 2g

Cholesterol: 38mg

Sodium: 811mg

Carbohydrates: 8.7g

Fiber: 1.9g

Sugar: 5.9g

Protein: 18.2g

Bacon & Jalapeño Soup

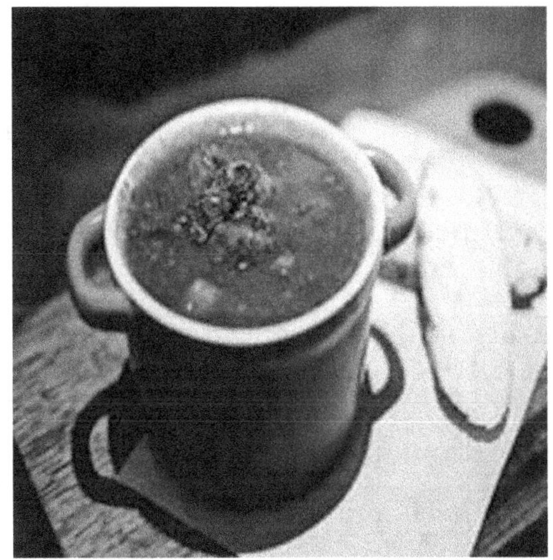

Servings: 2

Preparation time: 15 minutes

Cooking time: 22 minutes

Allergens: dairy

Ingredients:

¼ cup of unsalted butter

4 medium jalapeño peppers, seeded and chopped

1 small yellow onion, chopped

1 teaspoon of dried thyme, crushed

½ teaspoon of ground cumin

3 cups of homemade chicken broth

8 ounces of cheddar cheese, shredded

¾ cups of heavy cream

Salt and ground black pepper, as required

6 cooked bacon slices, chopped

Directions

In a large pan, melt 1 tablespoon of the butter over medium heat and sauté the jalapeño peppers for about 1-2 minutes.

With a slotted spoon, transfer the jalapeño peppers onto a plate.

In the same pan, melt the remaining butter over medium heat and sauté the onion for about 3-4 minutes.

Add the spices and sauté for about 1 minute.

Add the broth and bring to a boil.

Reduce the heat to low and cook for about 10 minutes.

Remove from the heat, and with an immersion blender, blend until smooth.

Return the pan over medium-low heat.

Stir in ¾ of the cooked bacon, cooked jalapeño, cheese, cream, and black pepper, and cook for about 5 minutes.

Serve hot with the topping of the remaining bacon.

Nutrition:

Calories: 549

Fat: 46.5g

Sat Fat: 24.6g

Cholesterol: 135mg

Sodium: 1900mg

Carbohydrates: 4.5g

Fiber: 0.9g

Sugar: 1.7g

Protein: 27.9g

Broccoli Soup

Servings: 2

Preparation time: 10 minutes

Cooking time: 15 minutes

Allergens: dairy

Ingredients:

4 cups of homemade chicken broth

20 ounces of small broccoli florets

12 ounces of cheddar cheese, cubed

Salt and ground black pepper, as required

1 cup of heavy cream

Directions

In a large soup pan, add the broth and broccoli over medium-high heat and bring to a boil.

Reduce the heat to low and cook, covered for about 5-7 minutes.

Stir in the cheese and cook for about 2-3 minutes, stirring continuously.

Stir in the salt, black pepper, and cream and cook for about 2 minutes.

Serve hot.

Nutrition:

Calories: 426

Fat: 32.9g

Sat Fat: 20.2g

Cholesterol: 104mg

Sodium: 1000mg

Carbohydrates: 9g

Fiber: 3g

Sugar: 2.9g

Protein: 24.5g

Yellow Squash Soup

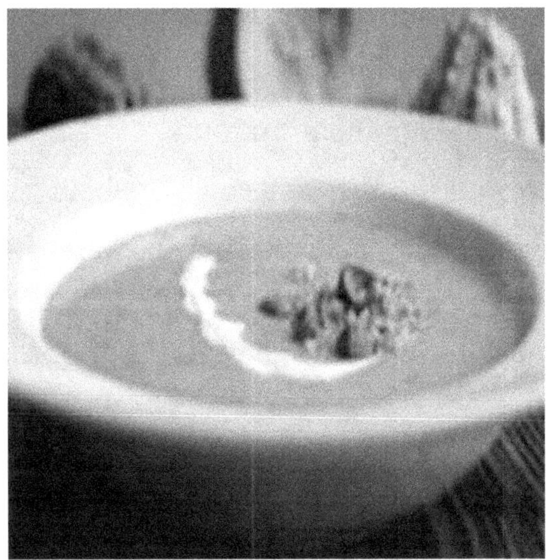

Servings: 2

Preparation time: 15 minutes

Cooking time: 35 minutes

Allergens: dairy

Ingredients:

2 tablespoons of unsalted butter

2 yellow onions, chopped

6 garlic cloves, minced

6 cups of yellow squash, seeded and cubed

4 thyme sprigs

4 cups of homemade vegetable broth

Salt and ground black pepper, as required

2 tablespoons of fresh lemon juice

4 tablespoons of Parmesan cheese, shredded

2 teaspoons of fresh lemon peel, grated finely

Directions

In a large soup pan, melt butter over medium heat and sauté the onions for about 5-6 minutes.

Add garlic and sauté for about 1 minute.

Add the yellow squash cubes and cook for about 5 minutes.

Stir in the thyme, broth, salt, and black pepper and bring to a boil.

Reduce the heat to low and cook, covered for about 15-20 minutes.

Remove from the heat and discard the thyme sprigs.

Set the pan aside to cool slightly.

In a large blender, add the soup in batches and process until smooth.

Return the soup into the same pan over medium heat.

Stir in the lemon juice and cook for about 2-3 minutes or until heated completely.

Serve hot with the garnishing of cheese and lemon peel.

Nutrition:

Calories: 115

Fat: 6g

Sat Fat: 3.4g

Cholesterol: 13mg

Sodium: 634mg

Carbohydrates: 9.8g

Fiber: 2.5g

Sugar: 4.2g

Protein: 6.6g

Chicken Soup

Servings: 2

Preparation time: 15 minutes

Cooking time: 25 minutes

Allergens: dairy

Ingredients:

2 tablespoons of butter

1 medium carrot, peeled and chopped

½ cup of yellow onion, chopped

2 celery stalks, chopped

1 garlic clove, minced

2 teaspoons of xanthan gum

1 teaspoon of dried parsley, crushed

Salt and ground black pepper, as required

4 cups of homemade chicken broth

10 ounces of cauliflower, chopped

2 cups of cooked grass-fed chicken, chopped

2 cups of heavy cream

¼ cup of fresh parsley, chopped

Directions

In a large soup pan, melt butter over medium heat and sauté the carrot, onion, and celery for about 3-4 minutes.

Add garlic and sauté for about 1 minute.

Meanwhile, in a bowl, mix together the xanthan gum, parsley, salt, and black pepper.

Stir in the parsley mixture, broth and cauliflower and bring to a boil.

Reduce the heat to low and cook, covered for about 15 minutes, stirring occasionally.

Stir in cooked chicken, cream, parsley, and salt and cook for about 4-5 minutes.

Serve hot.

Nutrition:

Calories: 442

Fat: 31.6g

Sat Fat: 18.5g

Cholesterol: 151mg

Sodium: 986mg

Carbohydrates: 11g

Fiber: 4.4g

Sugar: 4g

Protein: 28.4g

Meatballs Soup

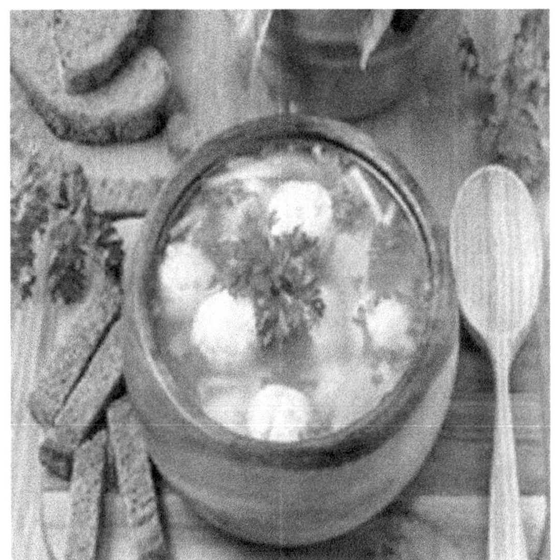

Servings: 2

Preparation time: 20 minutes

Cooking time: 25 minutes

Allergens: egg, dairy

Ingredients:

For Meatballs:

1-pound of lean ground turkey

1 garlic clove, minced

1 organic egg, beaten

¼ cup of Parmesan cheese, grated

Salt and ground black pepper, as required

For Soup:

1 tablespoon of olive oil

1 small yellow onion, chopped finely

1 garlic clove, minced

6 cups of homemade chicken broth

8 cups of fresh kale, trimmed and chopped

2 organic eggs, beaten lightly

Salt and ground black pepper, as required

Directions

For meatballs: in a bowl, add all ingredients and mix until well combined.

Make equal sized small balls from the mixture.

In a large soup pan, heat oil over medium heat and sauté onion for about 5-6 minutes.

Add garlic and sauté for about 1 minute.

Add the broth and bring to a boil.

Carefully place the balls in the pan and bring to a boil.

Reduce heat to low and simmer for about 10 minutes.

Stir in kale and bring the soup to a gentle simmer.

Simmer for about 2-3 minutes.

Slowly, add the beaten eggs, stirring continuously.

Season with salt and black pepper and serve hot.

Nutrition:

Calories: 288

Fat: 14g

Sat Fat: 4.8g

Cholesterol: 146mg

Sodium: 1171mg

Carbohydrates: 12g

Fiber: 1.6g

Sugar: 1.4g

Protein: 29.3g

Broiled Tilapia

Servings: 2

Preparation time: 10 minutes

Cooking time: 5 minutes

Allergens: dairy

Ingredients:

2 pounds of tilapia fillets

½ cup of Parmesan cheese, grated

3 tablespoons of mayonnaise

¼ cup of unsalted butter softened

2 tablespoons of fresh lemon juice

¼ teaspoon of dried thyme, crushed

Salt and ground black pepper, as required

Directions

Preheat your oven to broiler on high. Grease the broiler pan.

In a large bowl, mix all ingredients together except for tilapia fillets. Set aside.

Place the fillets onto the prepared broiler pan in a single layer.

Broil the fillets for about 2-3 minutes.

Remove from the oven and top the fillets with cheese mixture evenly.

Broil for about 2 minutes further.

Nutrition:

Calories: 185

Fat: 9.8g

Sat Fat: 5g

Cholesterol: 76mg

Sodium: 183mg

Carbohydrates: 1.4g

Fiber: 0g

Sugar: 0.4g

Protein: 23.2g

Creamy & Cheesy Steak

Servings: 2

Preparation time: 15 minutes

Cooking time: 1-hour

Allergens: dairy

Ingredients:

4 cups of heavy cream

3 tablespoons of Parmesan cheese, shredded

3 ounces of Gorgonzola cheese, crumbled

1/8 teaspoon of ground nutmeg

Salt and ground black pepper, as required

Pinch of onion powder

Pinch of garlic powder

Pinch of lemon pepper

4 (8-ounce) grass-fed beef tenderloin steaks

Directions

In a pan, add the heavy cream over medium heat and boil.

Then, reduce heat to low and let it cook for one hour, stirring occasionally.

Meanwhile, in a small bowl, mix onion powder, garlic powder, lemon pepper, salt, and black pepper.

Sprinkle the steaks with seasoning mixture evenly.

Preheat the outdoor grill to medium-high heat. Grease the grill grate.

Grill the steaks for about 4-5 minutes from both sides or until the desired doneness.

Remove the pan of cream from heat and immediately stir in cheeses, nutmeg, salt, and black pepper until well combined.

Place the steaks onto serving plates and serve alongside the creamy sauce evenly.

Nutrition:

Calories: 925

Fat: 65.6g

Sat Fat: 37.6g

Cholesterol: 390mg

Sodium: 563mg

Carbohydrates: 5g

Fiber: 0.7g

Sugar: 0.2g

Protein: 77.4g

Steak with Blueberry Sauce

Servings: 2

Preparation time: 15 minutes

Cooking time: 15 minutes

Allergens: dairy

Ingredients:

For the Sauce:

2 tablespoons of butter

2 tablespoons of yellow onion, chopped

2 garlic cloves, minced

1 teaspoon of fresh thyme, chopped finely

1 1/3 cups of homemade beef broth

2 tablespoons of fresh lemon juice

¾ cup of fresh blueberries

For Steak:

2 tablespoons of butter

4 (6-ounce) grass-fed flank steaks

Salt and ground black pepper, as required

Directions

For the sauce: in a pan, melt the butter over medium heat and sauté the onion for about 2 minutes.

Add the garlic and thyme and sauté for about 1 minute.

Stir in the broth and bring to a gentle simmer.

Reduce heat to low and cook for about 10 minutes.

Meanwhile, for steak: in a skillet, melt the butter over medium-high heat and cook steaks with salt and black pepper for about 3-4 minutes per side.

With a slotted spoon, transfer the steak onto the serving plates.

Add the sauce to the skillet and stir to scrape up the brown bits from the bottom.

Stir in the lemon juice, blueberries, salt, and black pepper and cook for about 1-2 minutes.

Remove from the heat and place the blueberry sauce over the steaks.

Serve immediately.

Nutrition:

Calories: 467

Fat: 24.3g

Sat Fat: 13.4g

Cholesterol: 123mg

Sodium: 473mg

Carbohydrates: 5.5g

Fiber: 0.9g

Sugar: 3.3g

Protein: 49.5g

Beef Curry

Servings: 2

Preparation time: 15 minutes

Cooking time: 3 hours 10 minutes

Allergens: dairy

Ingredients:

2½ pounds of grass-fed beef chuck roast, cubed into 1-inch size

2 tablespoons of butter

3 tablespoons of Thai red curry paste

2½ cups of unsweetened coconut milk

½ cup of homemade chicken broth

Salt and ground black pepper, as required

¼ cup of fresh cilantro, chopped

Directions

In a large pan, melt butter over low heat and sauté the curry paste for about 4-5 minutes.

Stir in the coconut milk and broth and bring to a gentle simmer, stirring occasionally.

Simmer for about 4-5 minutes.

Stir in beef and gain; bring to a boil over medium heat.

Reduce heat to low and cook covered for about 2½ hours, stirring occasionally

Remove from the heat, and with a slotted spoon, transfer the beef into a bowl.

Set the pan of curry aside for about 10 minutes.

With a slotted spoon, remove the fats from the top of the curry.

Return the pan over medium heat.

Stir in cooked beef and bring to a gentle simmer.

Reduce the heat to low and cook, uncovered for about 30 minutes, or until desired thickness.

Stir in salt and remove from heat.

Serve hot with the garnishing of cilantro.

Nutrition:

Calories: 753

Fat: 63.6g

Sat Fat: 33.6g

Cholesterol: 154mg

Sodium: 190mg

Carbohydrates: 5.8g

Fiber: 1.7g

Sugar: 2.6g

Protein: 39.4g

Beef Chili

Servings: 2

Preparation time: 15 minutes

Cooking time: 3 hours 10 minutes

Allergens: dairy

Ingredients:

2 pounds of grass-fed ground beef

1 yellow onion, chopped

½ cup of green bell pepper, seeded and chopped

½ cup of carrot, peeled and chopped

4 ounces of fresh mushrooms, sliced

2 garlic cloves, minced

1 (6-ounce) can sugar-free tomato paste

2 tablespoons of red chili powder

1 tablespoon of ground cumin

1 teaspoon of ground cinnamon

1 teaspoon of red pepper flakes, crushed

½ teaspoon ground allspice

Salt and ground black pepper, as required

4 cups of water

1 cup of sour cream

Directions

Heat a large nonstick pan over medium-high heat and cook beef for about 8-10 minutes.

Drain the excess grease from the pan.

Stir in remaining ingredients except for sour cream and bring the mixture to a boil.

Reduce heat to medium-low and let it cook covered for about 3 hours.

Serve hot with the topping of sour cream.

Nutrition:

Calories: 315

Fat: 13.8g

Sat Fat: 6.5g

Cholesterol: 114mg

Sodium: 90mg

Carbohydrates: 10.3g

Fiber: 2.6g

Sugar: 4.4g

Protein: 37.4g

Shepherd Pie

Servings: 2

Preparation time: 20 minutes

Cooking time: 50 minutes

Allergens: dairy

Ingredients:

¼cup of olive oil

1-pound of grass-fed ground beef

½cup of celery, chopped

¼cup of yellow onion, chopped

3 garlic cloves, minced

1 cup of tomatoes, chopped

2 (12-ounce) packages of riced cauliflower, cooked and well-drained

1 cup of Cheddar cheese, shredded

¼ cup of Parmesan cheese, shredded

1 cup of heavy cream

1 teaspoon of dried thyme

Directions

Preheat your oven to 350 F (180 C).

Heat oil in a large skillet over medium and cook the ground beef, celery, onions, and garlic for about 8-10 minutes.

Remove from the heat and drain the excess grease.

Immediately, stir in the tomatoes.

Transfer the mixture into a 10x7-inch casserole dish evenly.

In a food processor, add the cauliflower, cheeses, cream, and thyme and pulse until mashed potatoes like a mixture are formed.

Spread the cauliflower mixture over the meat in the casserole dish evenly.

Bake for about 35-40 mins.

Remove from the oven and let it cool slightly before serving.

Cut into desired sized pieces and serve.

Nutrition:

Calories: 411

Fat: 27.9g

Sat Fat: 12.2g

Cholesterol: 117mg

Sodium: 274mg

Carbohydrates: 9g

Fiber: 3.5g

Sugar: 4g

Protein: 32g

Dessert and Snacks on-the-go

Keto Bulletproof Coffee

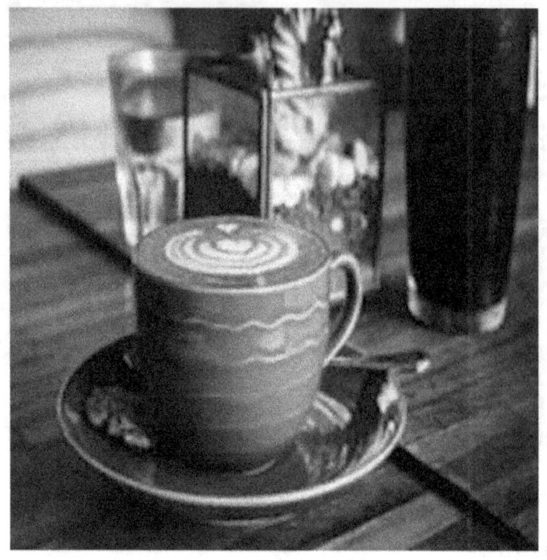

Serving: 1

Preparation Time: 5 minutes

Cooking Time: 0

Ingredients

1 cup of black coffee

1 tablespoon of grass-fed unsalted butter

1 tablespoon of coconut or MCT oil

1/2 tablespoon of heavy cream

1/2 teaspoon of vanilla extract

Directions:

Mix everything by hand or in a blender. Serve warm or cold! You can substitute almond extract for the vanilla or leave it out.

Nutrition: 255 calories, 28.5 g fat, 0 g protein, 1.0 g carbohydrates

Almond Butter Bulletproof Coffee

Serving: 1

Preparation Time: 10 minutes

Cooking Time: 0

Ingredients

1 cup coffee

1 Almond Butter Fat Bomb

Directions:

Brew your coffee as you normally would. Using your blender, blend the coffee and a Fat Bomb. Drink your coffee hot, or add ice cubes for iced coffee.

Nutrition: 300 calories, 31g fat, 7g protein, 4g net carbs

Raspberry Chia Pudding

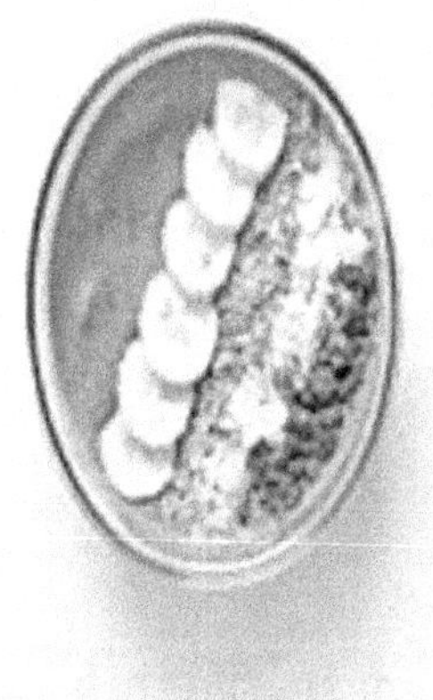

Serving: 2

Preparation Time: 5 minutes

Cooking Time: 5 minutes

Ingredients

1 cup of almond milk

1/2 cup of chia seeds

1/4 cup of frozen raspberries

1 Tablespoon of flaxseeds

1 Tablespoon of hemp seeds

Directions:

Combine all ingredients, mixing well, so the raspberries crush a bit. Store in an airtight container overnight. Enjoy leftovers within 7 days.

Nutrition: 642 calories, 50 g fat, 15.9 g protein, 8g net carbs

Raspberry Chocolate Fudge

Serving: 16

Preparation Time: 2 minutes

Cooking Time: 10 Minutes

Ingredients

1/2 cup of raw cacao powder

2 tablespoons of unsweetened dark chocolate shaved

2 tablespoons of Stevia

1/2 cup of coconut oil

1/4 cup of raspberries, mashed lightly

1/4 cup of almond milk

Directions:

Mix all ingredients until well combined. Prepare a 10" baking dish with parchment paper or plastic wrap, and carefully spoon the fudge mixture into the center. Using a spatula spread the mixture evenly into the baking dish, and covers with plastic wrap. Refrigerate for an hour, and cut into 16 equal pieces. Store wrapped in the fridge for up to one month.

Nutrition: 74 calories, 8.1g fat, 0.6g protein, 0.9g net carbs

Strawberry Chia Pudding Popsicles

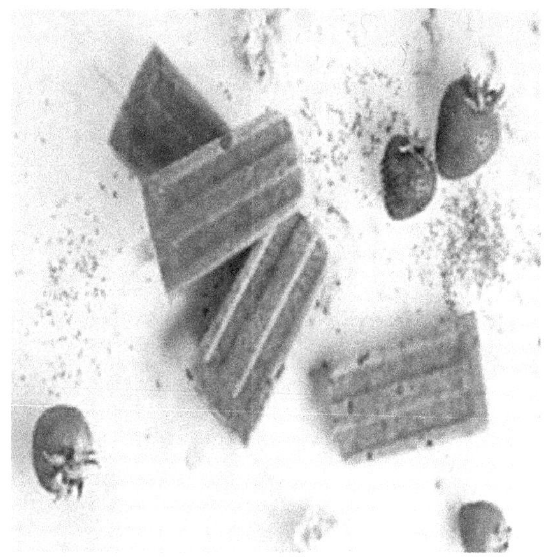

Servings: 6

Preparation Time: 4 hours, including freezing time

Cooking Time: 0 minutes

Ingredients

2 cups of coconut milk

1/4 cup of chia seeds

1/4 cup of frozen strawberries, thawed

Directions:

Mash the berries and chia seeds together. Stir in the coconut milk. Transfer the mixture to 6 Popsicle molds, and freeze for at least 4 hours. Popsicles will last in the freezer for up to 8 weeks.

Nutrition: 277 calories, 24.9 g fat, 5 g protein, 3 g net carbs

Almond Butter Cookies

Servings: 10

Preparation Time: 5 minutes

Cooking Time: 10 minutes

Ingredients:

3/4 cup of almond butter

1/4 cup of powdered Stevia or erythritol

1 egg yolk

1/4 teaspoon of cinnamon

Directions

Preheat oven to 350F. In a medium-sized bowl, beat together all ingredients until smooth. Roll the cookie dough into 1-1 1/2" balls, and lay them out onto a baking sheet lined with parchment. Press each ball down with a fork to form the final cookie shape. Bake 10-12 minutes, until golden brown and fragrant. Let the cookies cool completely before serving. Store cookies in an airtight container at room temperature for up to a week.

Nutrition: 98 calories, 10 g fat, 4 g protein, 1.4 g net carbs

Caramelized Onions

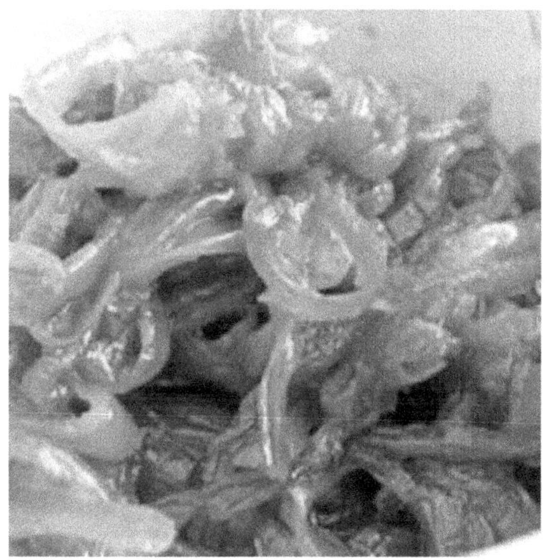

Servings: 8

Preparation Time: 10 minutes

Cooking Time: 65 minutes

Ingredients:

4 onions, sliced thinly

1/2 lb. butter

1 Tablespoon of salt

Directions

Melt the butter in a pan over medium heat. Add in the onions and the salt. Toss well with tongs until the onions start to cook down. Continue to cook, occasionally stirring, for about an hour, until the onions are brown and soft. Transfer to an airtight container and keep in the fridge for up to 4 weeks.

Nutrition: 225 calories, 23.1 g fat, 0.9 g protein, 3 g net carbs

Curry Mayonnaise

Servings: 8

Preparation Time: 5 minutes

Cooking Time: 0 minutes

Ingredients:

1/4 cup of mayonnaise

1 Tablespoon of curry powder

Directions

Whisk ingredients together until smooth. Store in an airtight container for up to 5 weeks.

Nutrition: 45 calories, 5 g fat, 0 g protein, 0 g net carbs

Green Tahini

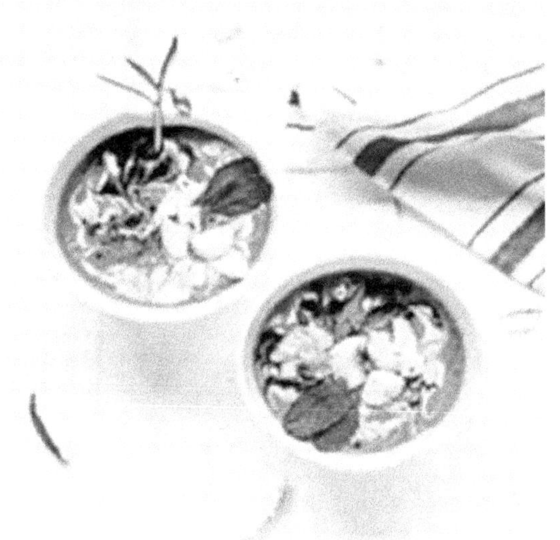

Servings: 8

Preparation Time: 5 minutes

Cooking Time: 0 minutes

Ingredients:

2 tablespoons of tahini paste

2 cloves of garlic

2 teaspoons of salt

1 tablespoon of olive oil

1 lemon, juice, and zest

1/4 cup of water

1/4 cup of fresh kale

Directions

In a blender or food processor, combine all ingredients until smooth. Taste and adjust seasoning as needed. Store in an airtight container for up to a month.

Nutrition: 43 calories, 3.9 g fat, 0.7 g protein, 0.3 g net carbs

Cheesy Fondue

Servings: 2

Preparation Time: 10 minutes

Cooking Time: 30 Minutes

Ingredients

1 cup of cheddar cheese, shredded

1 cup of gruyere cheese, shredded

1/4 cup of dry white wine

1 cup of heavy cream

1 teaspoon of garlic powder

1 teaspoon of salt

1 teaspoon of cayenne (optional)

3 stalks of celery, chopped into 12 equal sticks

1/2 red bell pepper, sliced into 8 thin strips

4 pickles, cut in half lengthwise

Directions

In a medium-sized saucepan, melt the cheeses and wine together over medium heat. Stir in the cream and spices, mixing well to combine. Transfer the finished sauce to a fondue pot, and keep warm. Arrange the veggies and bread onto a plate. Using fondue forks dip the veggies into the cheese sauce and eat immediately.

Nutrition: 376 calories, 32 g fat, 19.5g protein, 4.4 g net carbs

Green Bean Fries

Servings: 2

Preparation Time: 10 minutes

Cooking Time: 10 Minutes

Ingredients

24 green beans

1 egg

1/2 cup of parmesan

1 teaspoon of garlic powder

1 teaspoon of Italian herbs

1 teaspoon of salt

Directions:

Preheat oven to 400F. Fill a small pot with water for up to three quarters. Bring the water to a boil. Blanch the beans for 2 minutes, and immediately drain and transfer them to an ice bath. Next, beat the egg in one bowl, and combine the dry ingredients in another bowl. Prepare a baking sheet lined with parchment. Bread each bean by dipping it first into the egg, then into the cheese mixture. Lay the prepared beans on the baking sheet, and bake for 15 minutes until crispy. Store any leftover beans in an airtight container at room temperature, and enjoy within 4 days.

Nutrition: 113 calories, 6g fat, 9g protein, 2g net carbs

Seed Crackers & Guacamole

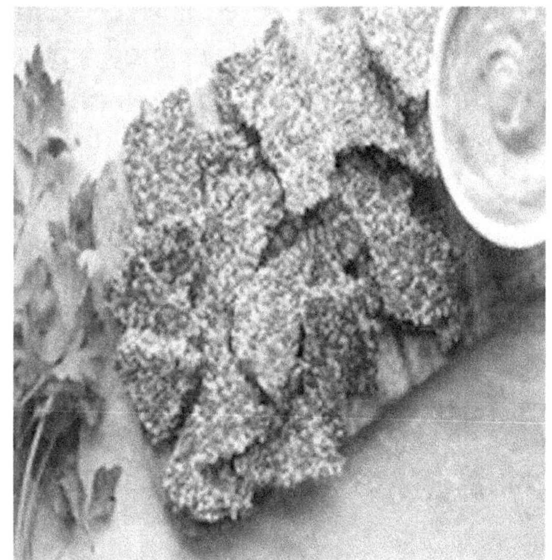

Servings: 2

Preparation Time: 10 minutes

Cooking Time: 45 Minutes

Ingredients

1/4 cups of chia seeds

1/4 cups of sesame seeds

1/4 cups of sunflower seeds

1/2 tablespoon of Italian herbs

1/2 teaspoon of salt

1 cup of water

1 egg

1/2 mashed avocado

Juice of half a lime

Pinch of sea salt

Directions:

Preheat the oven to 350F. Combine the seeds, herbs, salt, and egg in a bowl and allow the mixture to sit for 5 minutes. Line a baking sheet with parchment paper and spread the seed mixture evenly until flat. Bake for 30 minutes. While still warm, cut the seed mixture into 12 equal-sized squares. Flip the crackers over and bake for another 15 minutes. While the crackers are baking, combine all the guacamole ingredients in a bowl and mash until smooth.

Nutrition: 280 calories, 24g fat, 8g protein, 3g net carbs

Celery and Almond Butter

Serving: 1

Preparation Time: 2 minutes

Cooking Time: 0 Minutes

Ingredients

2 stalks of celery

2 tablespoons of almond butter

Directions:

Cut the celery into 8 equal-sized sticks and dip into the almond butter. For a more portable snack, spread the almond butter into the cavity of the celery stalk and pack in an airtight container for up to 24 hours.

Nutrition: 230 calories, 18g fat, 8g protein, 4g net carbs

Salted Macadamias

Serving: 1

Preparation Time: 5 minutes

Cooking Time: 5 Minutes

Ingredients

1/4 cup of Macadamia nuts

1 tablespoon of coconut oil

1 teaspoon of sea salt

Directions:

Preheat oven to 350F. Toss the macadamia nuts in the oil and salt. Lay onto a baking sheet, and bake for 5 minutes, making sure not to burn the nuts. Allow cooling fully.

Nutrition: 224 calories, 22g fat, 3g protein, 1g net carbs

Nordic Seed Bread

Servings: 12

Preparation Time: 10 minutes

Cooking Time: 30 minutes

Ingredients:

1 cup of almonds

1 cup of walnuts

1 cup of ground flax seeds

1 cup of pumpkin seeds

1 cup of sesame seeds

1/2 cup of ground macadamia nuts

1/2 cup of sesame seeds

5 eggs

1/2 cup of coconut oil

2 teaspoons of salt

Directions

Preheat oven to 325F. In a large bowl, whisk together the eggs, oil, and salt. Add in the seeds and mix well to combine. Next, press the mixture into a loaf pan lined with parchment. Bake for 1 hour and allow cooling fully before slicing. Slice the bread into 12 equal-sized pieces and wrap individually. Keep leftover pieces individually wrapped at room temperature for up to 4 weeks.

Nutrition: 369 calories, 31.5 g fat, 10 g protein, 5 g net carbs

Almond Butter Fat Bombs

Servings: 6

Preparation Time: 5 minutes

Cooking Time: 5 minutes

Ingredients:

1/4 cup of almond butter

1/4 cup of coconut oil

2 tablespoons of cocoa powder

1/4 cup of Stevia or erythritol

Directions

With a mixer or by hand, mix the almond butter and coconut oil. Microwave for about 30-45 seconds to soften, and then stir until smooth. Add the cocoa powder and the sweetener then stir those in and mix well. Pour into either silicone or mini muffin tins lined with papers. Stick in the fridge until firm.

Nutrition: 189 calories, 19.1 g fat, 3.2 g protein, 1.4 g net carbs

Mediterranean Fat Bombs

Servings: 6

Preparation Time: 10 minutes

Cooking Time: 5 minutes

Ingredients:

1/2 cup of cream cheese

1/4 cup of butter

1 teaspoon of dried oregano

1 teaspoon of dried thyme

1 teaspoon of dried basil

1 teaspoon of garlic powder

5 pieces of sundried tomatoes, sliced

3 olives, sliced

1/4 cup of parmesan cheese, grated

1/2 teaspoon of salt

1 teaspoon of pepper

Directions

Beat together the butter and cream cheese until smooth. Beat in the rest of the ingredients, making sure everything is evenly mixed. Prepare a baking dish with a bit of coconut oil. Spoon the mixture in and spread it evenly throughout the dish. Refrigerate for an hour, up to 6 weeks. Cut into 6 equal pieces.

Nutrition: 155 calories, 15 g fat, 3 g protein, 1.2 g net carbs

Chapter 7: Final Tips and Bits of Advice

Get a glass of water.

We often confuse thirst with hunger. This means that when we're thirsty, we reach for food, thinking it will satisfy us. What we really need is water. To drink more water, keep the water in front of you. For example, when you work, put the water bottle on your desk.

Measure your progress

Once a week or month, pull out the measuring tape, grab the scale, and write the new numbers down. Keeping track of your progress will help you stay focused and see how far you've come. Keep in mind that while you lose a lot of weight during the first few weeks, afterward, you might find out that you will lose about one pound a week. This is completely normal. If you want to measure by measuring tape, about one inch off your waistline equals about five pounds of body fat. You could also consider keeping a photo diary, where you photograph yourself topless in the mirror about once or twice a month. Apps like MyFitnessPal will help tremendously.

Get enough sleep

Sleep will help you make better choices. Getting better sleep will stop the stress from affecting your day-to-day judgments and generally make your life better. Lack of sleep also stimulates your appetite, meaning you'll want more food than normal. You won't feel satisfied, and you'll just want to keep eating. Take the time to get the best sleep, and take a break from the alarm clock once or twice a week.

Pick a Mantra

Did you know that negative thinking changes your brain's chemistry, and negative thinking attracts more negative thinking? Well, good news: positive thinking does the same thing. People really underestimate the power of positive thinking. Picking a mantra, something like "eat to nourish your body" or "90% kitchen, 10% workout," can help you reach your goals. Repeat it to yourself when you particularly feel down or like you're missing out.

Be Persistent

You need to keep going, even when it feels as if there is no progress being made. Plateaus occur after a while. Real change only comes with consistency. Real, slow-burning consistency. It can take a while to see real change, but it's pretty incredible when it does happen.

Stay Motivated

Staying motivated, especially when things like plateaus occur, is very hard. Hitting a plateau sometimes seems akin to hitting a rock wall.

Find a cheering squad: having a social circle that is supportive can be helpful too. Not only can they keep you on track, but they can remind you how far you've come and encourage you. Posting about your journey on social media is a great way to do this. Finding people who are also participating in the keto diet is a great find—mostly thanks to the fact that they'll be able to help you through the rougher parts of the diet. Social media is an incredible thing that enables you to connect with hundreds of millions of people overnight, many of whom are struggling with the same thing. Check out a Facebook group or the tags on Instagram. Just remember to ignore trolls, and vicious internet commenters with nothing nice to say.

Make Small Changes

Small habits change everything. Things like drinking more water and learning about nutrition are something that is never too late to do. And it would be nice if we could just jump into the keto diet without having to worry about completely changing your eating style. However, you might find yourself in way over your head, and all you want to do is eat a giant plate of French fries.

Cutting out foods you love can be tough. There is no shame in taking it easy, at first, and making small changes. This can be anywhere in your journey to a better you—things like taking a nice walk at lunch instead of eating at your desk and reaching for the veggies and guacamole instead of the regular bag of chips for a snack.

Making small changes benefits you over time because you're turning them into habits. You're replacing the bad habits with the good ones, and instead of depriving yourself, you're whittling them down. Some people out there have gone completely cold turkey, and that works for them, but that might not be for you. You might find yourself relapsing and craving carbs and junk more than ever—not because you want to eat it, but because your body is so dependent on it. Consider just cutting down on your habits and replacing what's in your fridge with the food you want to eat.

Don't Use Food as Rewards.

Rewards specifically imply that you've done something amazing, so why would you choose something that could set you back on your journey? An award should add to your journey, not make it worse.

What's the point of eating healthy for a week if you just plan on bingeing for a single day by eating whatever you want? Not only will you gain back all the weight you have lost, but you'll also knock yourself right back out of Ketosis and make the cravings for carbs and sugars worst.

Remember: that sundae you've been thinking about or the big pizza slice you've been eyeing will throw you out of Ketosis rather than being rewarding to you. It will only set you back, moving you right back to first base. Also, thinking of food as a reward can negatively affect your relationship with food by sending you the message that it's only something to be enjoyed on occasion.

Control Emotional Eating

We have all been there. We're bored, tired, stressed, and anxious, you name it, and we end up reaching for the foods that are not good for us. Things like our day-to-day lives can make us feel anxious and alone, and we often reach for food as a way to comfort ourselves. We also reach for food when we have nothing better to do. This needs to stop, not only because it will mess up our macro counting, but it is also not good for us.

Consider these helpful tips:

When stressed: soak in a bath, read a good book, meditate, or do some yoga. Find a healthier way to relax than chowing down.

Low on energy: Your first thought might be to pick up a snack, but if that's not doing it for you, take a walk around the block, listen to some energizing music, or take a short nap. Don't just mindlessly reach for more food—it's likely not the problem.

Lonely or bored: Call a friend and chat for a bit. Take your dog for a walk. Read a book or watch your favorite show on Netflix. Just keep your mind occupied.

Practice Mindful Eating

Mindful eating is when you're just paying attention to your food. You're doing nothing else except eating. This means the following:

• No distractions. This means no reading, no watching TV, no driving. This kind of mindless eating will only lead to overeating.

• Pay attention. Pay attention to your food. You should; you put a lot of effort into making it. If your mind wanders, keep your focus on your food. Think of it almost like a date that you have to impress.

• Eat slowly. It takes time for the signal to reach your brain that you're full. Politeness may have drilled into us that we have to eat everything on our plates, but don't feel too bad. It just means you have leftovers for later!

All in all, that's it! If you follow these healthy tips, you'll be burning those ketones in no time at all!

Take Help of Positive Affirmations

Positive affirmations are very inspiring. They fill us with positive energy and help in clearing away negative thoughts. You can read positive affirmations, listen to them on the internet, or recite them loudly. They help in every way. Positive affirmations keep your mind clear and give you the energy to sail through the bad times. They don't take much of your time, and you also don't have to remain dependent on others.

Share Your Goals with Your Family and Friends

Sharing such things with others is always difficult. There is always the fear of being judged on the results. However, there are always some people in everyone's life who don't judge. It can be your parents, partner, siblings, or close friends. Share your goals with them and the problems you are facing. Discuss with them the ways to get out of the problems. They can give you suggestions or at least lend their ears. Even letting it off your chest is also a great relief most of the time.

You will always have an assurance that there are people who really understand your efforts and are supporting you in them. You don't need to disclose your goals to everyone, but sharing them with some of your very close people is always a good idea.

Professional Help

Obesity is not a rare problem these days. In fact, it is one of the most common ailments now. Therefore, you can also get several professionals with whom you can discuss your problems and progress. You can consult your doctor and periodically review your progress. This serves two purposes. First, there will be a professional to guide you about the progress. You will get professional opinions on time about the problems you face on your way. You can get nutrition tips and also advice about the ways to improve the progress.

Support Groups

It is a cost-effective way to get help. Support groups can be your pillar of strength. Many people are suffering from the same problems. They are also going through the same trials and tribulations. They can prove to be a great help in case you need moral or mental support. Most people in support groups face similar problems, so your problems can be common. You can get the tips that worked for them. Such support groups can be of great help.

Keep the Atmosphere at Your Home Conducive

Most of the time, our surrounding atmosphere also makes our efforts difficult. For instance, if your fridge is full of carbonated beverages, fast food snacks, and munchies, it would be difficult to control the urge to eat. If people in your home are casually eating things all the time, you could start feeling punished and left out. You must explain your goals and make arrangements so that the process gets simpler and not difficult.

Maintain a Healthy Lifestyle

A sedentary lifestyle that doesn't involve exercise or physical activity is one of the cornerstones of weight gain.

If you're hoping to keep the weight off after you've stopped observing keto, you might want to consider adopting a healthier lifestyle to keep your metabolism fired up.

Daily routines that account for no more than 30 minutes of your time can be more than enough to keep that extra weight from creeping back onto your body.

Cardio exercises can be easy and practical for maintenance. Still, since you're probably consuming more carbs and proteins after keto, you might also want to incorporate some weight lifting into your repertoire.

Heavy lifting and high-intensity workouts that are demanding on your body will burn more calories not only immediately after the workout but also as you go throughout your day.

So, if you'd still be burning calories up to 8 hours after a jog, you could burn calories for as much as 24 hours after heavy weight lifting.

Keep Calories in Check

If you eat more calories than you burn, you will gain weight. That's just one of the basics.

So, if you want to make sure that you're keeping the weight off, you should be careful not to eat more calories than your body needs in a day.

Do you need to create a major deficit to achieve weight maintenance? Not exactly. Staying within the ideal limit can be good enough.

So, if your calculations tell you that you should consume a total of 1800 calories a day to meet your caloric needs, you can stick to that. You can create a minor deficit with your exercise or by taking out a small number if you really want to be on the safe side.

Eat Clean

Just as you're encouraged to indulge in healthy keto food, you should also make it a point to observe a clean diet once you're off of ketosis.

Healthy, whole foods that come as close to the source as possible are always the best. So try to avoid anything packaged, canned, or processed. Healthy food choices help improve your overall wellness and keep your body working in tip-top shape.

As a general rule, you should still aim to steer clear of junk food, sugary sweets and treats, and fast food since they never really provide any nutritional value whatever diet you might be on.

On top of that, you might also want to consider the way you prep your meals. Choosing healthy recipes that incorporate all the different essential food groups can give you balanced nutrition. Include vegetables and fruits into your diet, and make sure to eat just enough meat, along with your daily intake of carbs.

You might also want to opt for cooking methods that use less oil, such as roasting or boiling, to get the highest nutritional value from your chosen foods.

To make sure you're really investing in your health, it's also ideal that you consider taking multivitamins or supplements that can help fill in the gaps that might be present in your diet.

Even individuals who are particularly mindful of eating only healthy, whole foods are likely to miss out on a few micronutrients, so try to find the gap and fill it in with a trusted supplement.

Get Support

Weight loss and weight management are two tasks that are made easier with the help of friends - so make sure you get some well-deserved support.

Having someone with you who's out to achieve the same goals can make it much more difficult to fall off the wagon since you've got a little extra motivation.

What's more, working with a friend to achieve weight management makes it easier to get back on track if you find yourself straying away from your proper path.

Work out together, plan meals together, and keep each other updated on your success and even your failures. Don't be afraid to be honest with one another - failure to meet some of your new diet parameters shouldn't be shameful.

Aim to comfort each other during times of failure and uplift one another to get back on the wagon after a bad day. Being accountable to someone else is a great way to help you stay on track.

You might want to get support by finding online groups and forums where dieters discuss their progress. Social media platforms are an excellent example of places where you can find like-minded individuals on the same journey.

Applications for tracking your progress, meals, and exercise also have like-minded communities where you can share information on how your diet is getting along.

Maintaining a presence on these types of platforms makes it much easier to commit to your new diet. Herd mentality improves a person's resolve to stay on track, especially because many others can inspire you with their progress and personal experiences.

The ability to share information on your journey can also amp up your desire to keep going, so try to find people or communities that allow you to talk about how far you've come.

Conclusion

Your dedication to improving your health and losing weight is phenomenal since you have reached the end of this book. It is not an easy process to lose weight, but if you can maintain the guidelines you have learned in this book and stay motivated, your life will change in ways that you cannot imagine. You are on the right track to achieve both mental and physical health. Even though adjusting to eating a healthy diet after being accustomed to eating a lot of convenience foods is a challenge, you will feel the difference in energy levels that you will experience. You will look good and be safe from many of the common nutrition-related diseases and conditions, and on top of all of that, your quality of life will improve greatly.

All the answers to the questions you may have are included in this book to create an intermittent fasting plan. Eating the right foods and monitoring your progress when you first begin is the key to achieving success. Committing to your fast and learning which style is the best for you are all part of the process of incorporating intermittent fasting into your life. The next step is to practice intermittent fasting for at least thirty days to give it the time and opportunity to demonstrate that it can help you in your weight loss goals, improve your clarity, maintain better sleeping habits, and make better food and nutrition choices.

Once you begin following your schedule of fasting and begin incorporating each of the tips outlined in the book, you will achieve an increased appreciation of Intermittent Fasting and the benefits your body will derive from it.

It should have been informative and provided you with all of the tools you need to achieve your goals, whatever they might be. They can be weight loss, being more focused, building a better life—whatever! You should be able to walk away from reading this, knowing where you need to go and that you learned a lot.

The next step is to start the keto diet and keep going. It may be rough for the first few weeks, but it will get better. Track your goals, keep yourself motivated, and really embrace the idea of being a better and healthier you. Your body will be thanking you for years to come, and you'll feel so much better for it.

Remember: you are in control of your diet. You control whether or not you say no to foods that you know are bad for you. You are in control of the foods you stock in your kitchen, the foods you order at a restaurant, how much you eat— everything. You control what goes into your mouth, and you have a right to know what it is doing to your body.

From the moment you bought this book, you became a winner. You became a champion. Not everyone is brave enough to dare to change their nutrition and feeding methods in such a drastic way. Most people fear to fail, but what differentiates the normal people from the special people are the people who succeeded by getting out of their comfort zone, people that are disciplined and persistent towards reaching their goals.

Even if you are starting and find it really hard, or if you started but quitted, don't give up, keep pushing, keep trying and see amazing and unbelievable changes to start happening. This does not only apply to this diet but to everything in life.

Intermittent fasting helps you lessen body fat stores effortlessly in the entire body by changing the metabolism for breaking down body fat rather than muscle or sugar.

Intermittent fasting is an amazing concept not only for losing weight but also for gaining holistic health benefits.

It is free of cost and easy to follow. This book was intended to explain the concept of intermittent fasting and how it can be incorporated into daily life for the best results.

You can also get all the benefits of the process by following the simple steps given in the book.

Intermittent fasting is the best way to lose that bothering weight most naturally. Setting up a schedule is all you need, and of course, you need to follow it. Intermittent fasting has many forms and types that you can follow.

You can choose any type that suits you best. You can manage and hold the strings of your life through it. Is weight a bother to you? You can control it with your perfect diet schedule, even some keto diet plan in it. If not with diet, many other options are waiting for you for your consideration. You can opt for water-consuming plans, yoga, exercising, staying happy, mental stability, etc.

If you do not consider obesity as a problematic situation, you might end up piling yourself for the worst. There can be many greater problems waiting for you. Like diabetes etc., their stages might advance as well. You would end up spending a lot of resources and time on your doctor. Hence it is better to control it in the initial stage. You can gain control over yourself, over your mind, over your decisions, and how you want your body to operate. You need to control your diet. By that, it does not mean you cannot eat what you want to. You certainly can. But you just need to know the timings that you are allowed to dine.

The diseases that can cling to your body can destroy your life. Life expectancy rate can also be endangered. Women are also persistent in consuming fatty foods full of cholesterol, high fructose levels, high sugar levels, syrups, and Tran's fats even.

You can say goodbye to your obesity and see the difference in just a month. It is very helpful for you if you are lazy and tired of going to the gym. Stick to the plan by only being seated and watching a movie—no need for dieting. You need your essential proteins, but you need them at their time when your body requires them. You need to follow your body's needs rather than the love of your taste buds asking for creamy pulps all the time.

9 798618 084147